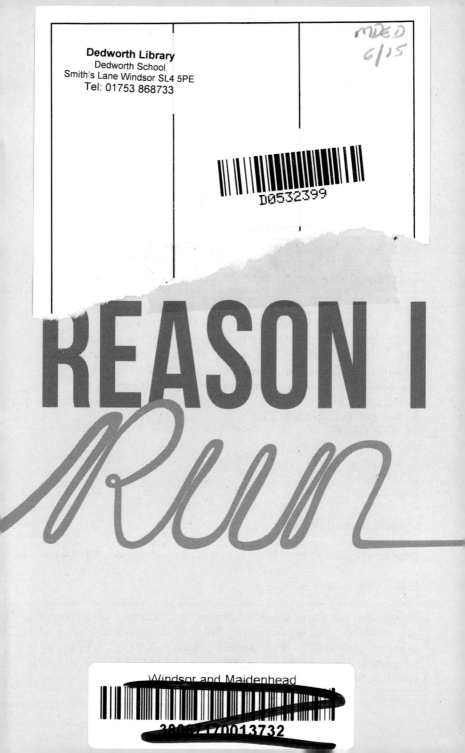

REASON I
Run

THE REASON I RUN

Copyright © Chris Spriggs, 2015

Summersdale Publishers Ltd
46 West Street
Chichester
West Sussex
PO19 1RP
UK

www.summersdale.com

Printed and bound by CPI Group (UK) Ltd, Croydon, CR0 4YY

ISBN: 978-1-84953-724-7

Substantial discounts on bulk quantities of Summersdale books
are available to corporations, professional associations and
other organisations. For details contact Nicky Douglas by
telephone: +44 (0) 1243 756902, fax: +44 (0) 1243 786300 or
email: nicky@summersdale.com.

THE REASON I

Run

HOW TWO MEN TRANSFORMED TRAGEDY INTO THE GREATEST RACE OF THEIR LIVES

CHRIS SPRIGGS

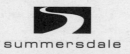

summersdale

Dedicated to my uncle Andrew and his family
And all those pursuing a world free
of motor neurone disease

FOREWORD

In my daily work as the chief executive of Motor Neurone Disease Association I never cease to be amazed by the acts of courage and determination shown by people living with this horrible illness.

MND is a particularly cruel condition, for which there is currently no cure. Although not common, it kills around five people every day in the UK – a third within a year of diagnosis. It can affect people in a variety of ways, including progressive weakness of limbs and eventually total loss of movement. Almost all will lose the ability to speak, meaning that communication of even one's most basic needs is impossible without the use of assistive technologies.

For people with fast progression they can notice worsening of symptoms every few days and this can have a significant impact on people's mental wellbeing as more and more of their former life is taken away from them.

Of course this inevitably affects the people around them, who find their caring responsibilities increase as they are trying to come to terms with the deterioration of their loved one. We know all too well the devastating impact MND has on families.

And yet. And yet.

In the face of this adversity – or perhaps in spite of it – people find a way to cope, carry on and see the positives. To find unusual and heart-warming ways to fight back.

Which brings me to Chris and his uncle Andrew.

This book tells the story of their sheer determination not to be beaten by MND and how a shared love of running created a very positive focus in both of their lives.

As a runner and a cyclist myself, I found this story both inspiring and uplifting. If you are a runner or you know someone living with MND or if you just need a good story about courage and the fight to live your life to the full, this is a book for you.

People with MND tell us they want more people to know about the disease. Help Chris and Andrew spread their vital message by reading this book and sharing their story: a story of hope and determination.

Sally Light
Chief Executive
Motor Neurone Disease Association

CONTENTS

I realise this is it! My feet on the puddled road, my hands clenching the wheelchair. I hear the sound of my breath, rasping and keen; and the sea, clawing at pebbles, sucking them back into itself. This is our moment, our chance. This is what we came here for. I grip my uncle's shoulder and say it as loudly as I can, above the chanting sea and the cheering crowds, 'This is it, Uncle Andrew, THIS IS IT!'

Brighton Marathon, 14 April 2013

FALLING...

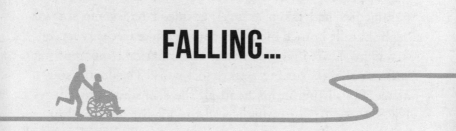

I collapse to the ground. A lady at my side gasps. A child points his finger at me. I look up and see the digital clock ticking... ticking... The finish line of the Beachy Head Marathon is within sight, at the bottom of a steep 60-metre hill. Beyond that are more Sussex cliffs with October sunshine spilling gold upon them, the horizon, and then who knows what? My uncle Andrew inspired me to attempt this race.

'It's one of the toughest in England,' he'd told me earlier in the year. It used to be his favourite race when he could still run. Right now it looks as if I won't quite make it.

Just a few weeks before today's race, an ambulance had rushed me from home to Warwick Hospital, its sirens waking my neighbours. That's when a doctor told me I might never run marathons again.

'We need to work out what's going on with your heart, Mr Spriggs.'

I may have looked over my shoulder to check with whom he was talking. This wasn't a conversation on first-name terms. It was serious.

'We think you may have had a mild heart attack,' he said, his hands lost deep in his pockets.

It appeared, from the electrocardiogram readings the paramedics had taken at my bedside, I had some sort of 'right bundle branch block'. It sounded like tree surgery, but it was my heart that was under examination. Apparently it wasn't ticking... ticking... like clockwork. The doctor stared at me as if listing in his head all the scans and procedures I was about to go through, and the kit list he would have to summon. The needles and swabs, the pads with wires, the pumps on trolleys. He sucked his lips, keeping some knowledge back, then turned abruptly and walked away. Then with a practised flick of his wrist he wrenched the cubicle curtains, causing them to screech along the metal pole like an impending car crash. He was putting me away for another time. I felt scared. I confess I was mostly scared my marathon-running days were over. I decided I shouldn't tell him I had 'one of the toughest in England' coming up within the next month, not until I knew more. Not until I knew what he kept in those pockets.

Lying here on the crumbling turf of the descent toward the finish line, my mind and body are in argument, millions of neurones gossiping possibilities about what is happening. The internal interrogation escalates: Why have you hit the ground? What's this about? Do you have the strength to continue? What's going on with your heart? Will you reach the finish?

Life is full of the unexpected. Not everything is as it seems.

So I have written this story. It's not 'Seven Steps to the Easy Life', neither is it a philosophy textbook, it's a story, and I accept it's my version of real events. Let me explain.

One day not so long ago my uncle Andrew was a marathon runner. It was part of Who He Was and What He Did. He ran distances longer than marathons, too, as if the finish line came too soon, so he'd go the extra miles. Literally, he'd just keep running. But then the lights went out on that phase of his life when something happened called motor neurone disease (MND). MND is a devastating life-limiting illness with no known cause or cure. Once it begins, there is no rewind button. The ability to move limbs and fingers and even control the tongue just fades. The strength to speak often closes down, until finally the body can't breathe. The end is coming way too early for him.

Uncle Andrew and I are ordinary men, easy to miss if you walked past us on the high street. We are not talented or spectacular runners, but we know the gifts that running brings. Our attempt at a marathon together, my uncle in the driving seat of a standard NHS wheelchair (because the illness means he can no longer run), and me behind him, pushing all the way, is the golden thread throughout this story. Our pursuit of 'one last marathon' for him became a joy for us in the context of unexpected and unwanted news.

One last marathon. But it didn't turn out that way.

So, who is this story for? It's for those who run, whether for a bus, or from the rain, those who huff and puff around the block, or are perhaps training for a marathon, or something else. There is a ridiculous pleasure to be found in escaping from under the duvet and daring to step out into the world. A strange metamorphosis occurs when you put one foot in front of the other, even when the way ahead seems unclear or beyond your capability. Running is hard; it can feel so alien in a comfort-obsessed society, but it often brings unexpected gifts. When you run, you change. Your world turns differently.

Running is one way that many people have reset their paradigm, their set of beliefs about themselves, learning to think differently about the chaotic and colourful circumstances in their lives. To begin to make sense of a world which is fragile, complex and sometimes nuts. Of course, running is not the only way you unfurl your sense of who you are in the world – perhaps walking up a mountain clarifies your perspective, or cycling restores your momentum, or swimming helps you reach for more. Whatever you most readily relate to, running is an activity most of us have done at some point, even if years ago down school corridors when no one was looking.

When you think about it, our language is rich with running idioms: the human race; pace yourself; the finish line; go the extra mile; hit the ground running; emotions running high; when your luck runs out.

Running is on our lips even if it's not in our legs.

This story is also for anyone who has ever faced a struggle that's threatened to squeeze the joy out of them. A loss, a heartbreak, a full stop in life where they've felt S.T.U.C.K. One of the messages of this story is that, however stuck you are, life is always moving, you are always changing. Your mind, body, surroundings, none of it is on pause. Amid struggle, you can find stillness. From stillness, flows clarity, then determination. And from determination, hope can be rekindled. With hope everything becomes possible.

There are questions woven into this story: Why do people run and what does it mean to them? What does coping with difficulty look like? How do people come together when tragedy tries to tear them apart? How do people start to make sense of the difficulties they encounter?

As philosopher Albert Camus wrote in *L'Étranger*, 'I finally learned that in the depths of winter there was in me an invincible summer.' To reach towards this 'invincible summer', we will listen to French firemen singing on the run, hijack a stranger from his seat during lunch hour, and race a Great Grandma at top speed around a medieval castle courtyard. We will search for a blacksmith in the snowfall of winter, chase after lorries in torrential rain and sprint along a wind-battered coastline with an air horn.

Why? Because now is not the time to give up.

THE SINGING
FIREMEN

*Although the world is full of suffering, it
is also full of the overcoming of it.*

Helen Keller

It happens at 3 a.m. on a June night. It's too warm to sleep.
I've wriggled so much the duvet looks like a massive reef
knot. News of my uncle's diagnosis has been on my mind for
a few months, but what happens in the night is not rational.
It's like this: one moment the idea is not there, the next it
consumes me. It arrives like an axe splitting a tree, sudden,
with no chance of reversal. I suddenly see that Uncle Andrew's
running days are over but his racing days do not have to be.

Lying in bed, staring at the ceiling, a solitary moment comes
back to my mind, an experience which stands out from all
the others the day I ran the Paris Marathon 2 years before.
A moment more prominent than the exuberance of the start

with 31,000 others on the Champs-Élysées, or the wine-quaffing relief at the finish.

Six miles into the race, as we entered the greenery of the Bois de Vincennes, I was overtaken by a group of firefighters. They were in full uniform, helmets reflecting the sun, running in a regimented way. In their midst they carried someone sitting in a wheelchair, strapped to poles either side and raised aloft, as if carrying royalty in centuries gone by. As they ran, they sang something happy, in French, all baritones sounding like an anthem of resilience. It was captivating, melodic and entirely unexpected. I didn't know the story of the young lady in the wheelchair, with physical disabilities that would prevent her from running in a playground, let alone 26.2 miles through Paris. I wondered what it must be like to be her, leading a life that could so easily be defined by what she couldn't do, and where she couldn't go, because of her condition and the inconvenience of a wheelchair. I didn't know the story, but it resonated.

'I realised as I looked down on the earth,' said Chris Hadfield, commander of the International Space Station, upon returning from 6 months of orbiting the earth and reflecting on what he'd learned, 'that there was no line between us and them. Just us.'

Is that what I witnessed in that French park? An erasing of the line between them and us, between can and cannot? Inspired by her and the firemen carrying her, I made a decision at that moment in the park. 'One day,' I said to myself, 'one day you're going to run for someone else like that.' Just without the uniform, big boots and jovial Gaelic singing. Then the moment of clarity was gone. The singing *pompiers* ploughed onward through the sea of runners, like a steamship determined on its course, and I was left in its musical wake, waves of runners lapping me up. I had no way of knowing then what that thought would become, when it would germinate, or the sad context in which it would come to life.

I forgot about that brief encounter in 2010 for the next couple of years; it had been like a whiff of fine perfume in a busy street, a passing revelation amid the pain of a marathon.

Now, it is nearly dawn, a riot of birdsong tells me. In my mind I see the singing firemen again, and although their anthem has faded, the charged emotion of the memory comes to the surface. I have no chance of sleeping now. I count down the hours until I can email my uncle with a suggestion. Although it's not a suggestion, it's a compulsion. A necessity, not a possibility, like how my wife, Hannah, feels about Ben and Jerry's Cookie Dough ice cream. I know how hard a marathon on two legs can be, but the seed of an idea sown on the run has penetrated my awareness in the middle of the night. I remind myself: my uncle's running days are over, but his racing days do not have to be. Each time I go over those words, determination sinks deeper, an anchor plunging into my depths.

I don't plan my email very well. I write it, delete it, rewrite it, the cursor dancing backwards and forwards. I am indirect and apologetic in tone. Thinking about what we've talked about together before, it's always been the everyday stuff. We've talked about life, not the flip side, not the reality of what his illness now means. I walk around the lounge, doing tiny circuits on the rug in case there is a message hidden in the weave.

Dear Uncle Andrew,

I hope you won't mind me venturing this thought. I was awake at 3 a.m. and it went round and round in my head!! If it's not something you want to consider then I fully accept that – and I at least wanted to ask, although I do feel a bit embarrassed asking... I wondered what it would be like if we both entered a marathon near to you (e.g. Brighton), and I pushed you round in a wheelchair, and we raised money for either the MND Association or Martlets Hospice, which I believe is near to you. OK, I know it's a bit mad, quite personal too, maybe it's far too early to contemplate it... I just wondered if you fancied a final marathon experience. I don't even know if Brighton allows such a thing.

Like I say, it was an idea at 3 a.m. and I've not been able to get it out of my head. Please do forgive me if I've stepped over a line with that suggestion. I just think there are more people for you to inspire, to hear your story, how far you've come and your resilience.

Have a think – and absolutely no obligation to give in to the idea.

Somehow the presence of the illness has interrupted the dynamic, unsettled the rhythm of a family relationship built on running. It wouldn't just be two runners: if he says yes, there will be a wheelchair to consider. Two's company, three's a crowd, but four wheels could cause mayhem.

I mention the Brighton Marathon for geographical purposes, just a 40-minute drive from his house, and there might be a chance the race organisers will allow wheelchair entrants. I also know my uncle has run the Rottingdean Off-road Marathon and the Downland Trail (30 miles), both local to Brighton. His decline in mobility coincided with the arrival of the first Brighton Marathon on the race scene in 2010, so it now hangs there, teasingly, as a major race he's never had the chance to take part in.

I give no consideration to factors like his mobility in 10 months' time. How about the comfort of sitting in a wheelchair for hours upon end? What about transport logistics? When is the closing date for the Brighton Marathon? (Less than a week away, as it happens.) Plus there's the small fact I haven't pushed an adult in a wheelchair more than 30 metres in over 30 years. Wonky shopping trolleys are my only reference point, and they didn't have adults in them either.

But I'm a big fan of Hope. Hope isn't dependent on what's going on out there, determined by fluctuations in the stock market, favourable sports results or evening news headlines. Hope needs a body to live in and a mind to nurture it. Those little sparks of light in our thoughts need looking after, need sharing with others who will fan them into flame, whatever time of the night they arrive. Hope isn't like daydreaming; it's dangerous when you act on it, because it changes you. And when you change, everything around you changes.

How do you prepare to race with a wheelchair for 26.2 miles? What does the body go through? What does the mind contend with attempting something you've never done before? Where are the limits? Maybe they're not where we think they are.

Time is not on our side. It's been a few months since I saw my uncle last, when the clues of his illness were evident in what he said, as we stood for a family photo in a restaurant car park.

My finger hesitates over the computer mouse. I press 'Send', put my hands behind my head, and sigh. The chair creaks at my back. I don't hear from him for 2 weeks.

A JOURNEY WITHOUT MAPS

One day can bend your life.

Mitch Albom

I had noticed it in the car park before I understood what it meant. Something different about my uncle's smile. It lacked the usual symmetry, as if hiding something sad. The change in his appearance over the previous year had been perceptible. The coming change in his circumstances was not.

Andrew is my favourite uncle, I think most people have a favourite uncle or auntie, secret or declared. Uncle Andrew was mine because with him I experienced those two things every boy wants and needs from the men in his life: To feel safe and to be respected. A kind of walking-talking 'everything's gonna be OK' message. Every kid wants that.

It had been a family day to celebrate my dad turning 70, but I walked away from the day with Uncle Andrew on my mind. Before leaving, we had gathered for the photo, my dad the birthday boy at the centre. Uncle Andrew stood at the edge of the group, next to me, and told me about the changes he was experiencing.

'I was out running a while ago and stumbled for no reason. I thought I'd just tripped so, you know, I got up again. But each time I went out, I was falling over. It kept happening.' He looked down, examining his feet, as if they were telling him something. These weren't the words of a new runner trying to work out how to run. This man has run along Kenyan beaches, through French vineyards, around Frank Sinatra's New York and Victor Hugo's Paris.

Here was a man who knew his legs well. How could this be?

His wife Sandra stood nearby as we readied ourselves for the photo. I listened to my uncle's words, but it was all the things not being said I tried to take in. He stood upright, hands in pockets, relaying his running accidents to me in a matter-of-fact way.

'I've got some… what do you call them?' he said, 'some new-… erm, new- neuro… logical tests coming up.' His stutter was like Morse code. A message to decipher.

A sad smile. Neurological tests. I knew something wasn't well in the world of my favourite uncle. It was the starting line of a life-limiting illness, which would dismantle his chance of ever running again.

For a while he had suspected the decline in his running performance was due to age. He'd written to me nearly 2 years earlier, just after I'd run the Paris Marathon with my wife and sister-in-law:

> I have been training for London, however for some
> time now I've lost a lot of speed (not that I had

much to start with!) I really struggled with the Cranleigh 21-miler 2 weeks ago, getting a Personal Worst by a long way. Old age rushes in! But I will get round and enjoy the day.

The clues were there.

The week following our meal and photo, my dad emailed to explain Uncle Andrew had been diagnosed with motor neurone disease. I confess I didn't know a single thing about it, so I began reading up about the illness, mainly on the MND Association website. I continued for 3 hours. The stories were incredible; of people facing the hurricane of an illness which steals the strength from their bodies, but who are determined to stay plugged into life.

I wanted to understand the facts, when I did they were not nice ones to know.

'It is impossible to convey in words,' says the MND Association, 'the overwhelming and devastating nature of a disease which in as little as a year can turn an active, able parent, partner or employee into someone totally dependent on others for the simplest actions we take for granted.'

MND is not an illness beaten in the same way that cancer can be fought and overcome, which in itself is no mean feat. I have numerous friends who have beaten cancer and there's plenty of celebration in their stories. Whereas cells multiply out of control with cancer, with MND they deteriorate out of control. MND is no respecter of age, ability or fame. Leeds United and England football player Don Revie, and acting legend David Niven both died of it. More recently it has affected the families of England cricketer Stuart Broad, television and radio personality Zoe Ball and climber Chris Bonington.

MND is an umbrella term for a range of ways the motor neurones in the brain stop working, as if packing up and going home early. The brain and muscles stop communicating with each other, so the muscles gradually and unpredictably stop doing what's required of them. The net result is an illness that eventually removes a person's ability to do the most basic things for themselves. Grip a mug of coffee. Scratch an itch. Say the names of those you love. Nip up the stairs. Tie your laces. Eat a biscuit. Swallow it. Breathe. MND takes the breath away.

There is no single test for the disease, it's based on the opinion of a neurologist and often other conditions have to be ruled out first. This means sometimes the process of diagnosis can take months, when every week is critical because it can be a fast-acting condition. Physicist Professor Stephen Hawking, who has MND, is an incredible anomaly. He was told by doctors he had 2 years to live, in 1963. He's just celebrated turning 73. But half of people diagnosed die within 14 months of their diagnosis.

The symptoms of the illness begin gradually and usually affect one side more than the other. Then it gets progressively worse.

'It is like a candle: it melts your nerves and leaves your body a pile of wax,' said Professor Morrie Schwartz, who became well known through his weekly encounters with author Mitch Albom, later encapsulated in Albom's popular memoir *Tuesdays with Morrie*. For my uncle, it is the weakness in his right shoulder that means lifting his fork and gripping the stair rail are becoming increasingly difficult. A cruel trade-off starts between exercising to strengthen the muscle but increased fatigue from doing so.

For some with MND, this disconnection between neurones and muscles predominantly affects the upper half of the body, noticeably making speech unclear (a condition known as dysarthria) and restricting hand grasp and arm lift. This is primary lateral sclerosis, which Professor Stephen Hawking has, and is the slowest form of the disease. When the neck and head are most affected, true for about a quarter of people with MND, this is progressive bulbar palsy. For others, it affects the lower half of the body far more, most noticeably the legs, known as progressive muscular atrophy.

I researched all this many times over. I memorised it. But when a friend asked me to explain it over coffee the facts had got lost in my head somewhere. I had to look it all up again. The form of MND I do know about is the one that's invaded my family and has a name, a face, a story.

My uncle has the most common and aggressive form, affecting about two-thirds of people with MND, known as amyotrophic lateral sclerosis (ALS), where both upper and lower motor neurones are damaged. Whichever form of MND takes up residence, the process is unique but the outcome the same. Its unpredictability is the challenge, with progression differing from person to person. MND upholds individuality while removing functionality. It is a journey without maps.

My uncle wrote to me a short while after his diagnosis:

> The disease progresses slowly but looking back I realise how things have deteriorated. A year ago I completed my last pub run (with the running club), but last week I had difficulty running for a bus! I can walk about 3 miles but generally feel very tired at the end of it, with aching knees and glad of a sit-down.

For 20 years as a long-distance runner, 3 miles has meant nothing to him. Now it's everything.

'Once he started running,' his son Paul told me, 'he was out all the time. I watched a marathon he was doing a few years ago and that's when I thought I'd like to run a marathon one day. My biggest regret is not taking up running earlier. I'm gutted I've not entered a race with Dad.' One day, father and son, running side by side. That was the hope.

'How did you feel when you heard about your dad's diagnosis?' I asked him.

'I was taken aback, to be honest. Like, I knew he'd been to the doctors, so I phoned him from work on my mobile. I remember speaking to him in a car park and not knowing what to say. The thing is, Dad was upbeat and said at least it wasn't cancer, meaning he wouldn't have to go through the uncertainty of whether he'd be cured or not.'

I try to imagine being on the end of that phone call. The silent gaps where thinking takes place, the spaces where words would usually be. 'I went back to work, trying not to think about it. But of course I kept thinking about Dad, then wondering how Mum would cope, then all sorts of stuff raced through my head. I felt really angry it happened to him, you know, as he'd always been fit and healthy. I was angry his grandchildren would miss out on doing things with their grandpa. To be fair it took a while to sink in. I couldn't believe it.' His voice level dropped, as if all the energy to cope was squeezed into those final words.

Now I sit in the quiet of my lounge, the night outside breathing calmly. I get out my black notebook, remove the elastic band, and find a new page to start jotting down the facts I've discovered:

Fact One. It's motor neurone disease, not motor neurons disease like I'd been mistakenly telling people.

Fact Two. A person's intelligence stays fully intact while the body dismantles itself.

Fact Three. Today five people in the UK died from it.

Fact Four. Any adult at any time can be diagnosed with it. It's twice as common in men than women, but it can be diagnosed in children too.

Fact Five. Around 5,000 people in the UK are living with MND today. All have names, talents and tantrums.

I pause and think.

Fact Six. The MND Association are the only UK charity providing support and care, campaigning for the cause and researching the illness. They loan equipment, like wheelchairs and walking frames, to maximise quality of life. They give financial support, and provide trained visitors to people facing MND, so they know they're not on their own. They have 90 branches run entirely by volunteers providing care. All this incredible work is going on in the background, every day, out of camera shot.

I turn to a new page.

Fact Seven. The cause is not yet known. 'There is a groundswell of medical and scientific opinion that MND is a disease that can be conquered,' says Professor Richard Ribchester. There is no cure yet, but that doesn't mean it's incurable.

The science is beyond me, to be fair, but at some point in the future, in a room full of microscopes and a rail of hooks on which hang white coats, someone is going to pick the lock of MND and uncover its mayhem-creating secrets. A world free of MND is a possibility. And if we crack the code for MND, that could help with understanding other neurological conditions. Am I naive? Having been an educator in schools on HIV-AIDS for nearly two decades, I've seen the incredible advances in medical treatment for that illness (but not yet the removal of the stigma). The transformation in life expectancy through antiretroviral drugs has been fantastic. I've spoken with teenagers and young mums in Ugandan clinics living with HIV. I've seen the need for advances in treatment to be made global. No, I'm not naive. But maybe I've got a responsibility to do what I can, where I am, with what I have. It's not what you say you believe, what you do is what you believe.

My pen tap-taps my knee, seeking a fault line through my defences. I walk to the window, and push back the curtain. I can't see the stars; there are too many street lights.

I flick to the front of my black book. There's a photo of a lady called Rosie, standing next to me, and a large yellow tent-trailer parked behind us, like an obedient guide dog. I retrieve the photo. The sharp edges of the picture curl in my hand as I remember the moment it was taken, just a few days after I'd run the Paris Marathon and seen the singing firemen.

Rosie Swale Pope ran around the entire circumference of the world. It took her 5 years, clocking up over 20,000 miles on foot, and getting through 53 pairs of trainers. She is the Imelda Marcos of the running world. Along the way she was confronted by bears, pursued by wolves, hit by a bus, struck by frostbite and chased by a man with a gun. He was naked. She also did much of it pulling a yellow trailer – her place to sleep as well as her storeroom – she affectionately called Icebird.

Running around the world was an idea that 'took her by the scruff of the neck' soon after Clive, her husband of 20 years, died in her arms, from prostate cancer.

'I knew with a passionate conviction I had to do something,' she says. So she did.

I'd spotted Icebird as I looked out my office window one day, parked casually outside a garage, looking as incongruous as an Eskimo with a spanner. I'd seen this iconic trailer in magazine articles about Rosie's adventure. A trailer crossing Siberia and the melted plains of Iceland. A trailer with a panoramic desert or a frozen landscape stretched out behind it, as if the dramatic backdrop was somehow attached to the rear of the trailer, not a garage forecourt on the Birmingham Road.

Next thing, I was having a cup of tea with Rosie by the roadside as she changed her socks. Light rain fell. Traffic fled past on its way out of town. She was part way through her '27 marathons in 27 days' challenge across England, pulling Icebird, who had just enjoyed a quick MOT. She asked me why I run. I got the impression she asked this question a lot, so I told her my reason. Then she looked up from pulling on her sock, smiled, leaned back and pulled from Icebird a black A4 notebook.

'I like that,' she said, 'yes, that's a good reason,' and asked me to write it down. I kept flicking through until I found a blank page, noticing the handwriting of many other people, using other words, describing other reasons they kept going. Novelist Haruki Murakami once remarked that whilst he only had a few reasons to keep running he had many more reasons to give up. 'All I can do is keep those few reasons nicely polished,' he said. Perhaps that's why Rosie kept a written list, to give her motivation a regular MOT. I found a fresh page, borrowed her biro, and leant the book on my knee to write the reason I run.

I'd hoped to join Rosie for the next section of her run that evening, as she still had a few miles to reach her marathon target for the day. But she needed time on her own to think. I recognised that if you've previously spent 5 years running around the world on your own, most of it through the vast wilderness of Siberia, you get used to your own company. She signed my copy of her book, *Just a Little Run Around the World*, posed for a photo in the drizzle and, like a rabbit down a hole, disappeared into her trailer. I figured she was done. But I'd caught some of her inspiration, and like a candle that shares its flame, it doesn't become less by giving itself away. That's when I decided to get myself a book and fill it with quotes and nuggets of inspiration. I made sure it was a black book, like Rosie's, but mine has a red elastic band around it. Rosie taught me the value of finding out why others make the journey they do, what powers them, with or without a trailer in pursuit.

I place the photograph back in the front of the book and write one more fact:

Fact Eight: There are many things which happen that we cannot control in life. Some are sad, cruel and unfair. But we can always choose our response.

MR HI-VIZ

Life is like riding a bicycle. In order to stay balanced, you must keep moving.

Albert Einstein

After 2 weeks of kicking myself for emailing such a ridiculous idea to my uncle, and at such a difficult time for him and his family as they absorb news of the diagnosis, he emails back.

> You are probably thinking you upset me with your madcap proposal, far from it, I am flattered you are willing to propose such an idea. I meant to reply before going on holiday and then forgot hence the delay in replying. My initial response to your idea for the Brighton Marathon was 'You're mad', however it has planted a seed which is nagging away in my head and I think worth investigating. Obviously there are lots of things to sort out but at this stage I am willing!

The elation of getting his agreement is tempered by the reality that we don't have a marathon race place. In fact, race entry is closed. And we don't have a wheelchair. Or any experience of putting the two together. Time is running out to make it happen.

Despite official entry for the Brighton Marathon being closed by the time my uncle replied, we approach Martlets Hospice, based in the Brighton and Hove area, who secure the last wheelchair place for us. We are delighted and relieved and Martlets become a fantastic support along the way. Like many hospices, they play an essential role in helping people to live life as fully as they can, right up until the end.

With my uncle's expectations raised, I need help learning to run with a wheelchair and to figure out some kind of training plan. I decide to hunt down somebody who can help. Our nickname for him was Mr Hi-Viz.

Occasionally I referred to him as 'the chubby bloke in the fluorescent orange top', when letting my kids know who I was talking about. He helps at a children's running event each month. I didn't mean it in an unkind way, but he stands out, wearing the top like skin. You can see him from 0.7 of a mile off.

One month, as the kids ran alongside the billowing white tape around the edge of the football pitch, our oldest son Caleb approached the finish line, leading the race. Then he tried out his new 'signature finish' and unleashed a double roly-poly along the grass, getting promptly overtaken to finish second. The post-race father-son conversation focused on the timing of roly-polies. Mr Hi-Viz came over to us.

'He's got something special, this one!' he said. That's when he emerged from the nickname and became Steve to me.

Steve is a car design engineer by trade ('I get to travel all over the world: Berlin, Detroit, Scunthorpe,' he told me) and a self-confessed latecomer to running.

'I took it up about six years ago because I'm a stress-head. I need my run. I go out most days, always with others.' We get talking some more at the kids' event and it appears Steve holds some secrets for what I'm hoping to attempt with my uncle.

Steve isn't just the proud owner of a hi-viz vest, he has a high-visibility personality to go with it. That's one of his secrets that could help me, but there's another more practical one.

He had been part of a team that pushed a lady in a wheelchair around the Kenilworth Half Marathon in our home county of Warwickshire. Just what I need. Somebody who knows something about this pushing-as-you-run thing. The lady had advertised for running helpers in the local paper, so he rocked up to do it. Steve and two other chaps had agreed to take on the duty and formed a wheelchair-pushing trio.

Having chatted in a muddy field at the children's running event, we swap contact details and arrange to meet up a few weeks later to run a 5-km parkrun together, and then get a coffee afterwards.

We are the muddiest customers in the cafe, tucked away in the corner, hot mochas in hand. The manager could easily follow our two sets of dirty footprints to track us down. As Vivaldi plays on the sound system, Steve talks me through his wheelchair racing experience, with lots of expressive gestures and rocking forwards and back. An apt drama to accompany Vivaldi's violins. I take notes in my black book, next to the facts I've jotted down about MND. I want to fill it with training tips and advice, but I also want to seize upon any insights into how people think when faced with difficulty.

'The lady was something special, she really was,' Steve tells me. 'After her newspaper ad, I went to her house. She opened the door and was dressed head to toe in a skiing outfit. You can imagine it! "Off we go," she says to me, and remember we'd only just turned up. On her way out she grabs a crash helmet, I mean a full-on crash helmet, and I'm thinking, "Like, how dangerous can this be?" My partner, Julie, had told me, "Whatever you do, Steve, don't just sign up," but she had this mesmerising presence. She puts the crash helmet on and loads herself up with dozens of energy drinks and gels. Honestly, you've never seen so many. But they weren't for us runners, they were for her. She's sitting in the wheelchair, I'm pushing her along, huffing and panting and really putting my back into it and she's happily chomping on energy gels, sat leisurely in the chair. She was something special, Chris, honestly.' Steve laughs and shakes his head.

The lady in question was Judy Woolfenden, a Kenilworth resident. She died 6 months after my conversation with Steve, at the age of 64, having suffered for more than 20 years from spinal muscular atrophy and a rare blood condition. Steve crossed paths with her more than once, also pushing her during a 100-mile ultra-marathon race as part of a team of six, completing the gruelling race in 29 hours between them. Judy raised hundreds of thousands of pounds for many UK charities and in 2007 received an MBE in recognition of her efforts for charity. Judy didn't look like an athlete, even with the ski gear, arctic down suit and crash helmet, but she didn't let her physical difficulties stop her from erasing the line and turning them into a story. Coast-to-coast wheelchair pushes. Eight marathons. Fifty-four hot air balloon rides. Judy was also the first person with a disability to tackle an

8-day dog sled ride through Swedish Lapland, a journey of 156 miles. Judy showed that making good things happen out of difficulties you experience is a mindset, not a luxury.

Steve's experiences with Judy were enriching, and her premature death was a sadness and shock for many.

'Judy was a real character, eccentric and so determined in everything she did. The words "can't" and "no" just didn't feature in her vocabulary,' he tells me.

I put down my empty cup, and the heavy clunk of it on the glass table sounds like a decision has been made. I lean back, notebook resting on my lap.

'People can really surprise you,' I say. 'So what advice would you give me?' I ask.

The hardest thing about pushing, Steve tells me, is trying to not kick the wheels as you run. His top tip is to attach my running watch to the handlebar – to save myself a crooked wrist. Useful to know. Vivaldi continues playing as Steve talks me through potential problems of, firstly, communicating to the back of a head (parenting is perfect practice, I believe) and secondly, navigating through the detritus at water stations. Thin NHS tyres and empty plastic bottles are not good road companions. You can tell he's walked the talk, or pushed the talk, as it were.

By the time Steve finishes a solo half marathon, I could be halfway round the course, for the second time, but he doesn't run for the clock or the medal. He runs to feel alive and straighten out his head. He has a zest for the road that Judy had, a belief that running is joy. He is now qualified as a running coach and has set up a group called 'Zero to Hero' to get others running, including teenagers and people in their plus-forties. He's animated about encouraging others, be they double-roly-polling boys or wheelchair-bound pensioners, wanting them to feel alive too, through the simple medium of putting one foot, one wheel, one smile in front of the other.

As we finish talking, Vivaldi gives way to the piano riffs of Jamie Cullum. A change of tune, a shift in rhythm. I look at the list of advice in my book. Which ones will I need? How will I work them into training? We go out through the automatic door. I hug Steve, hoping some of that hi-viz attitude to life rubs off on me. It's still 6 months to race day; it will have to last a long time. As we say goodbye, I don't realise that I too am about to have a wheelchair encounter which will require a crash helmet.

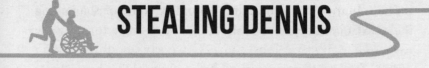

STEALING DENNIS

What one calls interruptions are precisely one's real life, the life you are being given day by day.

C. S. Lewis

I confess I am eyeing up his wheelchair.

My chat with Hi-Viz Steve about Crash Helmet Judy a few weeks ago has rattled my prejudice. I used to wonder what was 'wrong' when I saw someone in a wheelchair, rather than have any curiosity about their story. Why did I fixate on the wheelchair first and notice the person afterwards?

With my uncle's diagnosis, something's changing in me. This is why I'm staring across the coffee shop at the gentleman in his wheelchair eating his sandwich, little chunks of tomato escaping from the side, as he listens to his wife talk. I walk between the tables and arrive at their side like a waiter interrupting lunch.

'Sorry, but can I ask you some questions about your wheelchair?'

They look alarmed. I rapidly explain about my uncle and our marathon plan. I start asking about the seat, and that lever there, 'What does that do?' and the specially fitted bar joining the handles at the back – I need to know where he got it from. 'The NHS? eBay? Halfords?' These are the options I mention. They stay seated as I gesticulate, acting out invented semaphore, my arms trying to convey what I mean.

Then I grab the wheelchair handles and start pushing the gentleman out the double doors of the cafe into a busy car park.

'He's Dennis, I'm Sue,' shouts his wife hobbling behind me, waving her hand like she's hailing a bus. She has tendonitis. 'You can take him to the car if you want, I'll be glad for the break!' she says.

I pick up the pace, not knowing where their car is, weaving my way through parked cars like a slalom skier. I'm pushing a man I met 4 minutes ago, who is still chewing his sandwich, breadcrumbs clinging to his chin for salvation. And this isn't even on my training plan. Because I still don't have one. I narrowly avoid the concrete bollards and tip Dennis back to get him up onto the kerb. He splutters, so I jerk him forward. I let out a big sigh, he's a heavy chap and I may have started too fast. I'm often guilty of premature acceleration in races. I sprint down the pavement, all the way to the end, his comb over flicking up like a Mohican in the breeze, then turn and run back again. I have subconsciously mapped a route in my head of the car park. I wish I had my Garmin watch so I could measure the distance as a training run. I imagine seagulls and beach huts, sea air and the long iconic pier of Brighton, but in reality it's just a fast-food restaurant and a shopping-centre toilet block. This is hard work. We finally reach their car thanks to Dennis's hand signals, and I'm disappointed to discover I don't get a goody bag from Sue for my efforts. She opens the car-boot door and presses a button for a ramp to descend, and starts telling me their story.

'Oh, we've had quite a few months of it. I had a heart op last month, so we went on a cruise to recover. Then I got a call while we were in Sardinia to say my mum had died from a stroke. Then Dennis here (she points to her husband, just in case I'd lost track of who the man in front of me was) got an infection and we spent the last three and a half weeks of the cruise in a hospital. His muscles totally atrophied, hence the wheelchair.' She rolls her eyes.

'How did you cope, Sue?' I ask.

'Well, you do, don't you?' she says and looks at Dennis, who is still in shock from the fastest half-mile of his life. I'd call that the Traditional British Coping Strategy. Keep Calm and Carry On, which sometimes means Keep Quiet and Moan About It Later. If I remember, I will add this strategy into my black book.

Sue loads Dennis in his chair onto the ramp, as if tidying him away, tomato chunks and all, then gives me her phone number.

'Anytime you want to take him out, just ask.'

Dennis smiles as he gets lift-off, a snapshot of acquiescence. Sue leans towards me and in a hush says, 'When I've just about had enough of him I push him over the nearest cobbles I can find and watch his head wobble about like this.' She does an impression, we laugh. It seems like Sue has other coping strategies up her sleeve as she navigates her temporary troubles.

I wonder how my uncle will mentally adjust from two legs to four wheels. From being on the side of the super-able, to relying on someone else pushing him from A to B. Will he cope with cobbles and bollards and want to be fuelled by Italian bread and tomatoes?

My uncle emailed this week to say a friend of his works at Gatwick Airport 'doing passenger assistance', pushing people in wheelchairs from the terminal to the departure gates, which all sounds very ominous.

'We might need to look for something lighter, though,' he said, commenting that the airport wheelchairs are old and heavy. However, when it comes to it he gets one courtesy of the NHS. He's lucky it fits through his front door, as most people's door frames are too narrow, or they have steps up to their door. The reality is that none of us sets out to require a wheelchair one day. The arrival of an illness like MND means not only internal things change, externals change too. The height of the dinner table becomes impractical for a wheelchair in attendance. The upstairs bathroom becomes a nuisance to get to, so the cost of a stairlift has to be saved for. Driving responsibilities are gradually rescinded. Life is viewed from a height of 1.2 metres instead of 1.8. The words 'excuse me' are spoken on repeat down supermarket aisles, in cafes, along pavements. It can feel like the edges of one's life have shrunk.

With Uncle Andrew being a seasoned runner, he decides to get in some training practice sitting in a wheelchair. A friend of his, John, collects and takes him out so he gets used to bumping around on four wheels for hours at a time, covering some of the Brighton Marathon route together. 'It was just the flat part along the seafront,' my uncle tells me.

The Reverend Michael Wenham provides an insight, in his own memoir of living with the illness, into what it might be like for my uncle in a wheelchair in the marathon. Wenham describes a holiday in Italy 2 years after his own diagnosis of MND, where, however much he tried to sit comfortably, he bounced around as if on a trampoline, his arms falling off the armrest, feet slipping off the footplate and teeth rattling so much he couldn't talk. He suggests the only option is to give in and hope your driver notices the potholes in time. Then he nails the most important factor in the driver/passenger relationship: trust.

Given the look on Dennis's face after our spontaneous high-speed jaunt around the car park, I have a long way to go. I don't just mean 26.2 miles pushing my uncle, I mean being trusted. I need more practice. Oh, and to figure out a training plan.

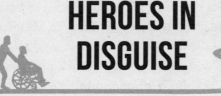

HEROES IN DISGUISE

My father gave me the greatest gift anyone could
give another person. He believed in me.

Jim Valvano

The first time I meet Mick, I nearly kill him.

A week after hijacking Dennis in his wheelchair and giving him the scare of his life, I find myself sitting in the same seat, in the same cafe. When it comes to pushing someone around a marathon in a wheelchair, specific research is required to get the training right. I tap a question into the *Runner's World* online forum on my laptop to ask for advice about how to best push and run at the same time. Ta-da! One medium cappuccino later I have responses from complete strangers from three corners of England. Some have experience of running with children's pushchairs, who advise on helpful postures; several others point me to one man. A chap called Mick Curry.

Mick is a man I've read about, the winner of a National Running Hero award with his son Phil, who has cerebral palsy and sodium valproate syndrome, which have left him without speech but with a great sense of humour. I have witnessed the duo in races I've participated in around South Warwickshire – the Stratford Summer Six, Kenilworth Half Marathon and Shakespeare Marathon. Mick looks ready to retire rather than run, but continues to push Phil, who sucks a plastic straw as they go, in his adapted wheelchair. They're an inspiring and intriguing pair.

After some detective work, I email Mick and get a one-line response from him, plus a phone number. I finish my coffee and get into my car to make the call. Twenty minutes later I arrive at his bungalow, in a cul-de-sac, which turns out to be only a mile away from the cafe. I grab my black book as I get out of the car.

I've come to hear his story, a story that would astound anyone facing difficulty. A story with answers to my questions about adapting to the unexpected in life, as well as how to make a wheelchair behave itself in top gear.

He opens the door and beckons me through the kitchen into the lounge.

'Don't worry about your shoes,' he says, as he takes a seat. With his thin-lined beard and two missing teeth in his bottom jaw, Mick might not look like the kind of man who has inspired thousands of people to run and not give up. But he is.

He chats about his day, then pauses before suddenly wincing. His face contorts, he stands and arcs his back, hand reaching for his hip. I wonder if this is a traditional greeting. I can't see anything wrong with the sofa he was sitting on, which appears to be new – after all, they've just moved into a new bungalow on a housing estate which is in the middle of a total overhaul. No, it's not the sofa, it's something else.

'I'm just recovering from an op,' Mick reassures me, breathlessly. 'Had some surgery... on my... lung, got hit by... a lorry twenty years... ago... and then fell out me loft... a few weeks back which... has triggered... the problem.' Phew. I was concerned for a moment that pushing a wheelchair was a major health hazard.

His painkiller regime is lined up on a table at the far end of the lounge. Pills with exotic names that probably taste foul.

'They make me a bit dozy, my friend, so if I... if I... er...' I sit attentively, like a student at his master's feet waiting for him to finish the sentence, but he never does. 'Er, where was I?' Right there on the sofa, Mick, right there.

It's all a bit surreal and I have to remind myself why I'm here and why I emailed him from the cafe this morning. How come this man, who I've never shaken hands with but have read about in national magazines, and who even has a race named after him and his son, has given up time to invite me round for coffee? A coffee that I had to make for myself, mind you.

'Thing is,' Mick said, 'you make someone a cuppa and it's too strong or too milky or... you know, blinking easier to make it how you like it, eh?' I got his point. He looked at me like I wasn't going to disagree. Not if I wanted my own coffee just how I liked it. I scoured the kitchen for sugar and milk until my eyes fell on a corner devoted to empty Lucozade bottles and cardboard pastry boxes. The treats in a runner's diet.

Many years ago Mick was a sub-3-hour marathon runner, a feat which requires closer inspection.

If you've run a marathon you'll understand the amount of training that goes into an achievement like that. 'I reckon I was doing about a hundred miles a week,' he says.

To run under 3 hours means running every single mile on average in less than 6 minutes 51 seconds. Mick individually completed over 20 marathons and was reaching his zenith when one day everything changed.

At the finish line of a marathon in 2002 his wife Dawn broke the news, 'I can't do this anymore, Mick.' Dawn, a sufferer of temporal lobe syndrome (a kind of epilepsy), had been pushing Phil around in his wheelchair, spectating and cheering Mick on at many of his races. Faithful, loud and true.

'I can't do this waiting around,' Dawn told Mick. 'Phil's been going crazy and it's too much for me. You either take him with you running or you pack it in.' There was the ultimatum. No wonder Mick had been speeding along in his races as fast as his legs would carry him, when wife and son were waiting at the other end desperate for him to get a move on.

What seemed like the end of his serious running career accidentally evolved into something that has taken Mick's life on a whole new course. A finish line became a start line. Dawn's suggestion, somewhat tongue in cheek, that Mick take Phil out running would of course require pushing him in his wheelchair. Phil can't physically run or self-propel his chair. He wears gloves and sucks plastic straws to prevent him 'chewing his fingers to pieces', Mick tells me.

'Pushing a grown-up son in a wheelchair is not easy or comfortable; it requires a lot of trust. Imagine running a marathon pushing a shopping trolley fully laden,' Mick explains. 'It's the front wheels that are the biggest problem – they go doolally, all over the bloody place they go.' Mick waves his hands as if they are fishes in the sea. I register this as a concern in my research and write in my book 'dodgy wheels'.

'Well, I can tell you now, I thought it was the end of things, so I had a long hard think,' he tells me. 'Would the wheelchair stand up to it? Would Philip like it? Most importantly, could I do this whilst pushing him? Running is hard enough at times, no matter what standard you are. This was make or break, all or nothing.' Mick reclines comfortably on the sofa and gazes up at the ceiling. I perch nervously, it's like we are connected, puppets on string, Mick leading the way.

'We started with a two-mile fun run, taking seventeen minutes forty-five seconds, moved up to a ten-kilometre race, clocking forty-six minutes, then tackled a ten-miler in a time of one hour forty-eight minutes.' He knows his times, that's for sure. 'The final test was the full marathon, where we achieved a time of four hours twelve minutes. This was fantastic, we were both loving it and, quite simply, having the time of our lives. The rest, as they say, is history.' Clearly Mick was starting from a very good foundation of running form and endurance, plus a talent for pace developed during 20 marathons.

They started taking on tougher, hillier races, mainly of half-marathon distance. They have now completed over 600 races including 41 marathons (the fastest being 4 hours 3 minutes, in Abingdon) and 300 half marathons (the fastest being 1 hour 43 minutes). The toughest race to date, Mick says, was Great Langdale in Cumbria, a half marathon they have completed twice, with a best time of 2 hours 45 minutes. All the adaptions to Phil's wheelchair have come from other athletes on their travels. Mick stresses to me that none of this would have been possible had it not been for sympathetic race organisers and the generosity of thousands of fellow runners. I figure a good supply of Danish pastries is also part of the recipe for success. I make a mental note to include a column on my training plan designated to pastry intake.

Mick says Phil is at his most content when he's on the move. His mobility is extremely limited so he is entirely dependent on Mick for all his needs. Looking after Phil through the years drove both him and his wife to mental breakdowns.

'She's no longer able to cope with Phil's extreme needs, but she's done a remarkable job over the years, I'm telling you, bringing him through his severe illness which almost cost him his life,' Mick tells me. There is a look of devotion in his eyes. His mouth opens and shuts, he runs out of words, his missing teeth like untold pieces of the story. This might be indicative of his admiration for his wife, or it might just be the side effects of his medication.

If you've not heard of MicknPhil then it may only be a matter of time before they roll off the tongue like fish 'n' chips, Morecambe and Wise, or any other great partnership. But there's a practical intelligence behind the trendy shortening of the 'and' between their names.

'The problem was when it was just me, I could enter a race solo. Easy, you know. But then when I tried to enter with Philip in the chair the organisers wouldn't let him in. Not at first. It was difficult.' This is a problem I will come across with my uncle in the months to come, with nearly every organised road race in the country stipulating no wheelchairs, buggies, skateboards, etc.

'Phil can't run. He can't talk. I've learned his signals now for him needing the loo in a race, or when he's wanting another straw to chew, but he can't run. So I started entering us as an all-in-one combo, MicknPhil. The computers couldn't tell the difference.'

MicknPhil are from a long line of defiant runners. In post-war Britain John Tarrant was a running legend, a long-distance folk hero, like Alf Tupper from the boys' comic adventure books. But like Mick and Phil, Tarrant knew what it was to be denied entry to races and became known to the world not as John Tarrant but simply as 'the ghost runner'.

Tarrant was banned for life from competing in athletics events by those in charge of the amateur running world, because he once received a small payment in a boxing match and was therefore deemed a professional. As a response Tarrant filled his rucksack with rocks and pounded the hills of the Peak District, becoming stronger, faster and more angry. In 1956, he arrived for a race in Liverpool, and stood as an unexpected extra alongside international marathon runners. Tarrant didn't look the part, wearing worn-out plimsolls and a shirt with no number. 'For over 20 miles no one could touch him; then, just as suddenly, he was gone,' wrote biographer Bill Jones.

For the next 2 years, 'the ghost runner' gatecrashed races all over Britain. Officials carrying his photograph would be left fuming when he hopped off the back of his brother's motor-cycle, took off his disguise near the start and ran his heart out, chasing the leading pack. The crowd urged on the man running with no number.

Tarrant was an honest man denied the chance to race. Like Mick and Phil. Like my uncle. For Tarrant it was a battle between the upper and lower classes. For my uncle it's a battle with his upper and lower neurones.

It's this same grit I see in Mick. Actions, not words. Not accepting a Them and Us world. Mick is a father just wanting to be in the race, with his son. To not be excluded or forgotten, denied or disadvantaged. Runners with no numbers wanting to play their part.

In 2008, MicknPhil's incredible journey was duly recognised when they won the Jane Tomlinson Heroes award, named in honour of the Yorkshire nurse who poured out her defiance running and cycling mile after mile, against breast cancer.

So how do people cope when they face difficult things? Mick Curry can add a few ideas to my list:

Adjust to a new reality, however unwelcome.

Reframe a problem as a new possibility.

Be willing to do something different, however unexpected or unprecedented.

Turn the question 'Can I?' into 'How can I?'

I write all this in my black book, next to a doodle of a fish and a dodgy-looking wheel.

* * *

Mick Curry becomes my point of reference when I want to find out about how to adapt a wheelchair so it can do marathons without impersonating that iconic four-wheeled scoundrel, the supermarket trolley. He knows his stuff. More importantly, I feel I've caught something of that indomitable spirit that over the last decade has seen MicknPhil travel the cities and rugged landscapes of the country in pursuit, not just of a finishing time, but of feeling really alive. Or as Mick puts it: 'Sometimes you just feel like... YEEEHAAAAAA!' and he was up from the sofa doing a merry jig, his toothless grin oozing joy, his back apparently recovered. It could've been the medication, but I think here is a man who has learned how to not yield to circumstances, but instead find a way through difficulty. He deserves every yeeehaaaaaa he can get.

Mick acts out a few things as part of coaching me in how to run a marathon with a wheelchair. For example, how to not roll backwards down a hill with it and how to stop it if you do; he acts out the difference between 'delirious' and 'tired' with great effect – putting me on the spot as to whether I know the difference. He uses facial expressions as if we are having a one-on-one game of charades. He wins, three-nil. Mick helps me see that running is many things. It is friendship. It is sacrifice. It is dedication. But it is also play.

After 2 hours of listening to Mick's story, I ask my burning question.

'Can I check out Phil's wheelchair?'

He leaps up from the sofa (he doesn't like sitting still) and takes me outside to the shed. I can see why he's got the impressive marathon time. He's out the door in a wink.

'Now, your standard NHS wheelchair comes in at about two hundred pounds or so, but ours got knackered. Gave up the ghost in some marathon or other, so I had to take it back to the start line and start the race all over again by myself. But this one...' Mick pulls it out to show me, like a fine vintage wine. 'This one was a few thousand pounds, but it's clocked a few miles since.' It looks very race-worn. 'Other runners clubbed together to buy it for me.'

I start rocking the wheelchair, hoping Phil in his absence won't mind. Mick explains why there is a dog lead attached to the undercarriage.

'If you go arse over you know what, you ain't got time to think – at least this way Phil won't go off without me.'

He's fitted bigger back tyres, plus a little wheel in the middle behind the seat a few inches off ground level.

'What's that for?' I ask.

'To stop it rocking too far back, of course,' he says. Then he suggests I take him for a spin around the half-built housing estate. As he settles into the chair, he describes how to get the rubber handle grips off the chair.

'They're damn useless once your hands are sweating, so dip 'em in boiling water, they're only glued on and the NHS won't mind.' I assume he means dipping the grips in boiling water, not my hands. 'Feel free to train with us anytime,' he says. 'You've got plenty of time.' I do the sums, there are less than 5 months to go.

What I considered to be a gentle incline in my car when I parked 2 hours ago, I now perceive as something imported from the Alps.

'How heavy... are you... Mick, if you... don't... mind me asking?' I gasp. He's as light as he looks, but this is tougher than my car-park circuit with Dennis.

Mick has a typical ectomorphic long-distance-running physique, so there's not a jot of fat on him, but it's an effort pushing him 20 metres. Even with Mick's genius idea of having four mountain-bike handle grips added, it feels like the chair has a life of its own and that it wants to continually rock backwards.

'Come on, son, push... POOSH, go for it!' Mick says. He's the front-seat passenger, I'm the back-seat driver. 'Take me up the hill,' he taunts.

I stagger up the hill as fast as I can, face parallel with the ground, my legs stretched out behind. Mick believed I was in good physical shape when he asked me for my running track record and personal-best race times. I'd come prepared for the questions.

'I ran Chester Marathon a few weeks ago in three hours eleven minutes, my best time so far,' I told him. Mick tilted his head as I answered, doing a calculation of some kind.

'OK, you're not too bad then,' he said. But credentials and credibility are not the same thing.

I grip Phil's souped-up wheelchair and remind myself of Hi-Viz Steve and Judy Woolfenden in her crash helmet. I grit my teeth and push harder, using as much gluteus-maximus muscle as I can.

'Hey, watch OUT!' Mick yells, arms in the air, hands vibrating as if I've plugged him in. I veer onto the raised pavement with a jolt to avoid the oncoming construction lorry. A builder leans out the window looking down on me, frowning and making gestures I won't sketch in my black book. What he sees probably won't make any sense, but who cares what he thinks? Unless he thinks I've stolen a gentleman from the local day-care centre and reports it to the police.

But I'm high on caffeine and pulsating with the inspiration of Mick's story. For now, that's enough to make it up this hill without killing him. Just. The real test will be finding out what it's like pushing my uncle in his chair. If I can't control him, we haven't got a hope.

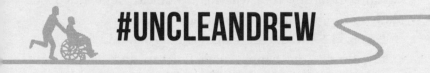

#UNCLEANDREW

Look up at the stars, not down at your feet.

Stephen Hawking

It sits on the drive, like a child on the naughty step.

After running 9 miles solo through stark winter countryside as part of my long training run, I arrive at my dad's house, and there it is. Uncle Andrew's wheelchair. I still don't associate my marathon-running uncle with a wheelchair. I'm here to collect and push him around, so to speak, as a practice for the marathon. He and Auntie Sandra have come up from Horsham in Sussex to Warwickshire to stay on a rare weekend without snow.

My training plan is starting to take shape. I'm still recovering from having run well in the Chester Marathon, where I had knocked 14 minutes off my previous best marathon time. So the plan is to do a long run of at least 10–12 miles each weekend to maintain stamina through Christmas; a hilly run of an hour (about 7 miles) and two shorter fast runs each week; and then to run with anything or anyone in need of a push whenever I get the chance, Dennis-style. I will average about 30 miles a week until February when it will have to go up a gear to nearer 50 miles a week. If my body permits.

We pose for photos outside the house. My dad, his wife Elizabeth and my Auntie Sandra all click away. I am in shorts, sweating from my run, whereas my uncle looks kitted out ready to climb Mount Everest. Click-Click.

'This is like a wedding!' laughs Auntie Sandra.

'Yes, we are the happy couple!' I say, and put my arm around my uncle's shoulder. The net curtains of the elderly neighbours twitch.

My dad and uncle Andrew look like brothers, even with 7 years between them, my dad being older. They had another brother, Graham, the one they both looked up to as kids, not just in age and height but in adoration too. My dad referred to Graham as his best friend, until tragedy struck when Sergeant Graham Spriggs was killed, aged 21, in a night-time collision involving two RAF planes. A young life suspended among clouds. Later that day had come an uninvited knock on the door of the family home. News from people in uniforms. Then hushed voices in the house. Uncle Andrew was 10. A family story that wasn't ever talked about.

We start our practice run. 'I'll take you through the village,' I say, 'although it doesn't have many sights.'

After more than an hour of running I'm warmed up, but I remember my recent encounter when I nearly got Mick run over by a lorry, so I keep it steady. We cross the busy B-road and go through the council estate, then on towards my sister's house. As we pass, I give a little wave to their windows, curtains still drawn. I tell my uncle about my sister's forthcoming cake sale to raise awareness and sponsorship for our race. We continue past my kids' school, gates padlocked, then towards my house. We've timed it just right.

My wife and her sister, Ruth, up from London for the weekend, and our three kids are all waving frantically from the upstairs window, knocking on the glass as if trying to escape. So many waving and wriggling bodies in the context of one window frame. It's like a massive passport photo, arms across faces and everyone vying for a view. Click-Click.

I switch from being self-conscious, looking like I've stolen a man from a bus stop, to being proud of what we are doing and why. We both wave, my uncle with his left hand, the one that still retains some strength for the time being, and then we carry on our way.

As I push, my uncle talks. It's the thing I enjoy most on this, our first and only training run, hearing more of his story. I had just pointed out where the Esso garage used to be in the village, now a supermarket.

'Yes, I spent my working life with Esso,' he says, 'I was always on the retail side. I guess you'd call it Area Manager these days, but it was different then.' He talks me through various office moves and how colleagues got him into running, helping him to lose weight, having been eating too well living in hotels all week.

'It was just after I started working at the new office in Leatherhead, having had two years in London. Some colleagues were going running at lunchtime so I joined them, building up the mileage as I went. Twelve months later, having said I never would, I did my first half marathon at Barns Green.'

Running with others is an important component for Uncle Andrew, being part of something bigger.

'We would do a four-mile loop at lunchtime, but I never ran all the way until the third or fourth time,' he says. A while later a colleague suggested doing a marathon.

'No way, that's just too far to run!' my uncle had replied. He chuckles as he retells the story, as if still surprised about what those lunchtime runs led to. One small choice defined his next 20 years.

He went on to run 46 half marathons and 36 marathons, plus three races longer than 26.2 miles, raising thousands of pounds for various charities, especially Chase Children's Hospice near to where he lives and from whom he got a special award of recognition. He started running in his forties, so that's a marathon (or longer) every 6 months. He's done great things, but the ability to do great things is temporary.

We start going up another hill in the village. My breathing quickens, my stride shortens. In fact, if you want to escape our village the only way of doing so is via a hill or a sharp incline over a bridge. I'm doing my best not to huff loudly. I extend my arms and put my head down.

'What about your proudest moment?' I ask, leaning towards his ear.

'Proudest moment? That's a difficult one,' he says. 'I was proud to finish Seven Sisters, which is now the Beachy Head Marathon, an off-road beast of a race. Really tough one to do. I finished it nine times. One of the toughest ones in England.' He pauses as if reliving the ups and downs of such a testing course. We cross the busy road and I tip the chair up onto the pavement, safely across to the other side.

Seven Sisters. My mind reverts to the first time I came across that phrase, one night at Scouts, when I was barely a teenager.

But it didn't refer to hills. I don't know why it's been stored in my brain all this time. A movie replays in my mind.

'You won't need your torch, just your eyes,' Skip said, his breath taking shape in the cold air. 'You have to look carefully, OK, just to the right of that one there,' he said, arm outstretched like a salute. Skip was one of my scout-troop leaders, a former fireman who, in an accident, had lost his ability to smell 'in the line of duty', he'd say. He said having no smell had advantages, and proved it, always volunteering to sort out the Portaloos at camp, which gave him hero status amongst the troop. Perhaps the loss of smell meant he channelled extra powers through his remaining senses. Skip was someone who wanted to help you see stuff, but what he was pointing to was so very far away. Clouds moved across, obscuring the place where his index finger was aimed like an arrow. Clouds travelled as if in a rush, the sky cleared and then I saw them. A fuzzy patch of stars.

'D'you see them?' he said. 'D'you see them, now?' as if repeating the question would help my eyesight.

A tiny moment, which now carries significance. The Seven Sisters are not striking or dramatic; in fact, only six are visible to the naked eye, but that evening they became my favourite constellation. Under their proper astronomical name, the Pleiades, they feature in Greek mythology, the Bible and stories of North American tribes. The Japanese call them Houki Boshi, meaning 'dabs of paint on the sky', and the Aztecs called them 'the gathering place'. They became my favourite constellation, not because of their legendary or spiritual status, but because it sounded like they were hanging out together.

Seven Sisters: a family who need each other.

It's only now I discover my favourite constellation shares its name with a set of hills on the Sussex coast. A series of seven undulating peaks, a roller coaster grooved into nature, and part of the route of the Beachy Head Marathon. They challenge the knees of any person walking them, but some people don't walk them, they run them. They feature somewhere after 20 miles along the course, meaning they're exactly what your body doesn't want at that point in the race.

'The race includes an immediate two-hundred-foot incline from the start,' my uncle says, 'and there's always a solo bagpipe player at the top of a hill, not sure why.' Within the coming year he will have persuaded me to give the race a go, and I will experience the chalk paths, the 300 steps, the 14 gates and the ridge-top trails where the wind is so ferocious it fills you like a sail. Running through the South Downs National Park there are checkpoints with chunks of Mars bars and Danish pastries and strumming folk bands. The views out to sea are expansive, especially from England's highest chalk sea cliff, Beachy Head itself, famous for the tragedies it's witnessed. It's a race that tests your capability, stamina and awareness. An adventure which fills your vision and satisfies your senses. No wonder it was the first thing which came to his mind when I asked my uncle the question. It had been his first off-road marathon, and 12 years later his last ever marathon on foot. That last one was also his slowest 26.2-miler ever, taking him nearly 6 hours.

'It's the sort of marathon where you just turn up and do the race, no hassle, no hype,' he says. 'My first time, it had been raining all week and poured down on race day. I didn't have any of those, you know, proper trail shoes you get these days,' he said. 'I was slipping and sliding all over the place, visibility was so poor I didn't realise how close we were to the cliff edge as we ran up and down the Seven Sisters hills.'

I take note to keep away from the edge of the pavement now as we scoot along, picking up speed.

'Mind you, the free jacket potato and fruit salad afterwards were very welcome.'

He had even entered the race the year it clashed with his twins' twenty-first birthday. His twins, Paul and Jo, confess to not being impressed with the standard of their dad's dancing at their party that night, when he stayed up until the early hours, having been up since the previous early hours that morning to run the marathon. It's not easy to dance well after running a trail marathon in just under 5 hours. It would look like a world-class performance compared to how he would dance now.

I don't know what Skip would make of the Seven Sisters hills. I think he'd prefer the version in the heavens to the earth-bound ones, but the Beachy Head Marathon is an experience where you have to pay attention to all that is before you and around you. You spend as much time looking down as looking up.

'I knew when I ran it for the last time,' my uncle says, 'it would be my last ever marathon. It was so tiring. But then you never know what life turns up for you.'

Is that why my uncle recommended it to me? A reminder we are a family who need each other?

'What else are you proud of?' I ask.

'I was pleased to run the London Marathon ten years in a row and proud to finish under four hours for the first time. Oh, and I was proud to do a personal best after fourteen years, in Paris. And… and… I'm proud to have raised money for different charities. Also, finishing the Steyning Stinger off-road marathon six years in a row was brilliant, with a PB (personal best) of four hours twenty-six the final time. I even got a shot glass as a race memento from there.'

Asking for his proudest running moment was like asking a father with six children to choose his favourite. Perhaps resilience – that ability to face adversity and overcome it – is rooted in a multiplicity of experiences, relationships and know-how, not just one crowning achievement.

I ask about the final time he ran the London Marathon, with his eldest daughter Sarah.

'I knew my running style had changed and it would be my last. Still, I managed to beat her by ten minutes! I never expected Sarah to do a marathon; she was never keen on running as a child. But then neither was I.'

We reach the top of the hill, the tough part done.

'What about your worst race then?' I have to strain my ears to hear him speaking into the cold wind.

'Again, it's difficult. One of my first tough ones was London in 1996, which was my third attempt. I felt in really good shape but it turned hot and at halfway my head was down and I was barely plodding. I finished in four hours twenty-nine minutes actual running time. The moral of the race?' He poses the question and leaves it there for me to mull over. I'm wondering if the moral is to not take up running. Think how much hassle could be avoided.

'The moral,' he says, finally, 'is you have got to do decent long training runs!' He speaks like a head teacher making his point firmly. 'When the time came to enter for the next year, I decided that poor performance could NOT have the last word. Later in 1996 I joined a running club, the Horsham Joggers, and I was lucky to get one of their club places to run the London Marathon in 1997, even though they didn't know who I was. I did track work and structured training and my performance improved. The following year I finally cracked four hours.'

Uncle Andrew speaks highly of the support and enthusiasm of his running club, with whom he is still in contact. He also took part in the Horsham Round a few times, a run of about 28 miles organised by the club, which could be tackled in teams or solo.

'I did the whole thing twice, with club mates at a similar pace, it was a very sociable run along bridleways and footpaths.'

We run towards the hamlet of Broom over a humpback bridge, crossing above the busy A46. I wave at vehicles driving beneath us. We must look suspicious to them, an apparent theft of an OAP being rushed away at high speed. This is the tricky bit: pushing one-handed and waving like the Queen. I hadn't practised this.

I had expected the problem to be the front wheels going doolally upon reaching a certain speed, but they behave themselves. I had anticipated my hand-grip to feel awkward, but the padded weightlifting gloves I'd purchased are working fine, even if they do cause my hands to resemble those of a coal miner for 3 days afterwards.

Although I experience no issues with one-handed wheelchair steering, it is more of a problem twisting the nozzle on my hydration pack one-handed, or consuming my GU chocolate gels one-handed, or even waving one-handed, because two-handed waves look a bit, you know, zealous. These are the issues. Wheelchairs, I decide, were definitely designed to be pushed by people with two hands.

'Do you still drive?' I ask him.

'Yes, my feet are fine. I saw my consultant last week and he didn't mention it. My right hand is getting weaker though, so I'll have to keep an eye on that.' Before the year is out driving will become another addition to the list of easily assumed functions that have to be packed away. I find this out from Auntie Sandra.

'He used to ask me who was driving as we got ready to go out,' she says, 'but then he just stopped asking.'

'What about occupational care and visits?' I ask him.

'Well, I've had a physio recommend certain stretches, an occupational therapist visits occasionally to assess the house and my mobility, and an MND nurse comes about once a month. They've all been excellent. I've not needed much nursing until now but obviously things will deteriorate.'

It's the reality of the disease, a gradual unplanned sequence of setbacks, from which there is no return. But his racing days are not over. I feel determined about this, sensing the same defiance shown by John 'the ghost' Tarrant, the man who ran despite being excluded.

Today, as my uncle tries to keep his toes warm and endures my heavy breathing from behind, I wonder what the perfect run is like. I think today is a perfect run, because, just like the perfect kiss or the perfect pudding, it's one I don't want to end too soon. On the other hand, if it never ended, it would end up not quite so pleasurable; but to be absorbed for the moment *in* life itself, *is* life itself.

We head through Broom and a short downhill section. There isn't much traffic, just the occasional dog-walker. As I push, every step feels an effort. My legs are starting to ache, given I've run more than a half marathon in total this morning. I suspect a couple of blisters have appeared, but I've enjoyed it. I rarely run with others, it's often a solitary thing for me, me in my moving bubble alone with my wandering mind, so this has been unlike any other run.

We pass the Royal Life Saving Society headquarters.

'What would make a perfect day for you?' I ask. Uncle Andrew is quiet for a few moments. I can feel the strain on my arms. I can hear the solid tyres whirring. I clench my teeth. Each step is like striking a tent peg into the ground.

'Historically,' he says, 'a perfect day would've been a good walk in the country with good weather, maybe a pub lunch. Now I'd say it's spending time with family, especially my grandchildren. I want them to have positive memories of me.'

Time. Something we're told to manage. To not waste. To make the most of. Perhaps it's not just spending time, perhaps it's also investing it. A life-limiting illness shatters the universal illusion that we are in control over the time we have. We have today. Who knows what tomorrow brings? That doesn't mean live for today regardless of consequences. If that were the case, we'd never put the washing on or pay the credit card. But to live today fully, to not hold back, to offer all that we are.

I consider the beautiful ordinariness of my uncle's perfect day, not littered with meeting the rich and famous or visiting wonders of the world. Just the chance to be with people he loves, to be fully present, here and now. Presence before Absence. To breathe it in. Today may just be the greatest day of our lives because it's the One Day we have for sure.

I save my most personal question until last. We've completed 5 miles together, my legs feel heavy given the miles I did before collecting him. There are still a couple of miles until home.

'What was your reaction to hearing you had MND?' I ask.

THE REASON I RUN

'When I was told it didn't come out of the blue, actually.' He talks in a level tone. 'Before I went to the doctor for the first time I'd read an article by Chris Woodhead, *The Sunday Times* educational correspondent, who has MND. What he described was similar to things I was experiencing. I guess that planted the seed, so when I first went to the doctor I asked him outright, "Is it MND?" He gave a vague answer. When I met the consultant he said he couldn't rule it out. When the diagnosis was finally confirmed, it was what I expected.'

'How did you feel?' I ask. There's a pause. I can't see his facial expression as we bump along the pavement.

'I was calm and rational. That was a year and a half ago and hey, I'm still here!' he says, throwing his left hand up from the wheelchair handle. This must be a sign he trusts me if he's not even holding on.

We pull up briefly by the side of the road, opposite a pub, for me to adjust my empty hydration pack. There at my feet, in a puddle, is a five-pound note. I pick it up.

'That'll help our sponsorship,' I say. Had it not been nine o'clock on a Sunday morning we might have taken a diversion to the pub, a perfect run followed by a perfect pint.

On the move again, I tell my uncle of the time I was running a couple of years previously, wondering what to get my wife for her birthday, when I found a neatly folded fifty-pound note looking unloved by the side of the road. I picked it up and looked around to see who'd dropped it. But I was alone. I sprinted home with it and a few days later bought my wife a dress with it.

'Running brings the most surprising things your way,' I say. My uncle laughs.

We surge up the final steep hill, I'm determined to run all the way, then I turn into the road where my dad lives. Our family are waiting, more photos are taken, before I run another mile home. Later in the day, having eventually totted up 7 miles together in 1 hour 15 minutes, an envelope falls through my dad's door. On it, in the wobbly handwriting of a pensioner, are the words 'To the runners' charity'. In the envelope? Fifty pounds. If we'd known our training run would be so lucrative, we'd have planned more together.

That was our one and only training run, me pushing my uncle for the first time. But the truth is my uncle had been pushing me for 7 years. Not in a wheelchair, but through his running example and as a coach when my own running journey began. This is a story which starts where another one ends.

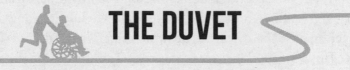

THE DUVET

*Before we can see properly we must first
shed our tears to clear the way.*

Indian proverb

My mum died on a Saturday, wearing a lilac nightie. It was
5.24 p.m. and cloudy.

She returned home from the hospice to die, her final wish.
She'd lost her hair through chemotherapy but the nightie
made it safely back home with her.

In those final days I drove to my parents' house to squeeze
out every last drop of time together. Perhaps I felt guilty about
all those years I didn't tidy my room or do the washing-up. I
accompanied her up the stairs to her room. Thirteen carpeted
stairs took 3 minutes to climb, each stair creaking as I
followed her, a woman of 59 years trapped in a 90-year-old's
body. The doctor said she had a matter of days to live but 99
per cent of my brain didn't believe a word of it. It switched
off to protect itself, to conserve energy for later. Emotionally,
I was holding my breath.

'You're a good boy, aren't you?' she said, as I helped her get ready for bed. She peeled off her clothes, in awkward movements. I saw her puny arms, skin unequally wrapped around bones, revealing where strength once was. She sat on the end of her bed, in disposable pants. My mum. The one within whom my own life was crafted, in her underwear. I helped her unravel the lilac nightie so it fell over her head. I sorted her pillows and said a prayer, all the while juggling my anger against the disease with wondering what I'd have for tea. This was my face-to-face introduction to cancer, aware my own life was coming apart by its impact. Yet there was little I could do but help my mum get ready for bed.

I tucked her in, then leaned over. I wanted to reach in and rescue her, make her like the mum I knew before the cancer, like the one in the photos downstairs. The mum who patted the back of her head, always conscious of how her hair looked. Strangely, after the chemotherapy robbed her of it she took to having a wig like a child with a new bike. On, off, and then back on again. The wig looked fantastic on her. The mum who started telling one story and ended up telling five stories instead, none of them related. My mum hosted all the unfinished stories in the world.

The mattress squeaked as I sat down. I closed my eyes and felt the tender weight of her hand in mine. There were no wires now, the connection was pure relationship and memory, not technology or hospital machines. I stroked the back of her hands, her bony fingers, noticing the contours of her knuckles, like the Derbyshire Peaks where she'd grown up. Years later I can still recall those sensations. All that hand cream over the years produced the softest hands. Perhaps it's not just the hand cream, but also the mothering and the giving that moulded hands like these, and the facts that my mum was a physiotherapist and chiropodist. Hands are like libraries, stories crammed into them, full of memory, like the fingers of a master pianist reciting Rachmaninoff. Oh, the stories hands can tell.

I rested my hand on the stubble of her hair, feeling the pulsating warmth in her head, blood rushing, heart pumping, still doing what it had always done. Defiance, tucked in under a lilac duvet.

'It can take your body. It can take your appetite. It can take your will to live. But it can't take away your friends and the people that love you,' she used to say about the cancer. I admired that bravery, for whenever she said it you could notice in her eyes the downright stubbornness of the woman that is, was, my mum.

My dad was doing his best to rest after an emergency hernia operation and I tried to figure out how life was for him. We were in this struggle together, yet the most distant we'd ever been. Lonely, not Alone.

During those closing days of her life, speculation abounded regarding the cause of the 7/7 London bombings a few days before. Our family sorrow was playing out in the shadows of national tragedy; a footnote to a Bigger Story that summer. Just another cancer statistic in 2005. Of course, I knew there were people all over the place facing similar scenarios, many far worse. My mum was just one of 3,617 women to die from ovarian cancer that year. One of many to experience the 'silent killer', because the symptoms are similar to other less serious conditions, like irritable bowel syndrome. For mum it was the persistent bloating, looking pregnant as she lay on the sofa. The pelvic pain. The feeling full so quickly. By the time the jigsaw of symptoms was clear, it was secondary cancer speeding in the direction of her bones and brain. Everywhere I drove Coldplay's 'Fix You' was playing on the radio but no amount of crying seemed to fix anything, tears hurtling down my face like Olympic sprinters. The tears stung. It would be more than a year before they soothed.

I'd had enough of cancer. My mum was going through treatment at the same time as my best friend David. It was David who called me from the other side of the world whilst he was on holiday when he knew my mum only had days to live. There were long silences on the phone between our words. He told me what I might expect. To make as much of the time as I could. To be strong, but also that it was OK to not always be strong. I knew he was drawing on his own reserves of experience. This wasn't textbook-answer stuff, this was a friend being alongside, even from the other side of the world.

Perhaps my loss was tame by comparison to others, but having a parent you love removed from your life is like an emotional hijack. There are no labelled diagrams showing you what will happen next and what to do. Sometimes loss mounts up so fast, a conveyer belt of heartbreak and worry, like when you're packing your shopping away and the checkout person is going too fast and you can't open enough plastic bags to pack it all away neatly (heavy items at the bottom, etc.) and you just want to hit a STOP! button. PLEASE JUST STOP! Sometimes life is like this, leaving you out of breath, thoughts half-packed, half-spilling over. Loss disorders you.

I watched my mum, knowing I was losing her. Nobody could reach her. I watched her sense of presence being pulled away as if over a cliff edge, my arms not long enough to keep her. I wanted to believe that God would do something, make it better right there and then. But he didn't, no matter how much gesturing and swearing at the sky and standing with my hands surrendered on my head. I didn't lose my faith then, but it changed. It migrated from Certainty to Curiosity. Loss helped me relinquish control of needing answers. Clouds came, clouds passed, but the permanence of the sky stood fast. I think my faith became both strong and fragile, depending on the amount of caffeine in my bloodstream at any given moment.

Her eyes were like tunnels, a strange glow, light from elsewhere. She was there but not there, being tugged into another world. Morphine a bridge to help her make the journey. Being around death is strangely fascinating. You notice things about life that are at other times obscured. The looming darkness of death shoves life into its finest and brightest perspective.

I dragged myself along on the journey of 'my mum and the cancer', naively hoping the clouds would hold back their threats. But I saw what ovarian cancer did, up close, how it robbed strength, dismantled dignity, made hair fall out. I hated it, but the years since her death have helped me feel a strange kind of gratitude for that awful lesson in death.

Those moments of quiet presence together helped me through a year of bereavement.

I edged away, my mum peeping out from the top of the duvet cover. Eyes unfocused. Skin paled. She joked a few nights before how the colour of her nightie went really well with the duvet and I think she was chuffed by this, fashion conscious even on her deathbed.

My wife joined me at the bedside. My voice cracked as I said my last ever words to my mum, words I must have chosen, as if I knew I wouldn't ever see her conscious again. Words that poured with the sound of goodbye: 'Sleep well, my beautiful.'

Our family all stayed the night, my brother Mark pouring red wine and reciting poetry aloud in the kitchen. We were walking through the valley of the shadow of death in style. A nurse from Shakespeare Hospice visited and brought kindness, then the vicar came, and brought listening ears. Peace rested heavily in the house like coastal night-fog, obscuring the precipice we were about to encounter. There was no foghorn. Death came quietly.

The following day was Saturday. At 5.24 p.m. my sister noticed my mum's breathing was shallow. We hurried to her side. Held her soft hands. Let her go.

This was no bomb blast in a big city, wreaking havoc and devastation, demanding attendance of dozens of emergency vehicles. There was no shattered glass or lost limbs, this was just a gentle slipping away under a heavily creased duvet. Death comes in many different costumes, but in the end it's never in disguise. You recognise it upon arrival.

At my mum's funeral I waited outside the heavy doors of the church building, the weight of her coffin resting on my shoulder, as 'Benedictus', from Karl Jenkins' *The Armed Man*, played inside. My brother gripped my arm, a shot of reassurance as we carried our mum in together, as if to say, 'We can live with this, bro, we can get through this.' It's true. We can live with it. We can get through it. But I didn't feel that at the time, as I tried not to buckle under the responsibility of it all. It felt like an audition, waiting off stage, feeling despair like a hammer wanting to Tap. Tap. Tap me into the ground, and bury me forever.

We walked down the aisle, in first gear, and placed the coffin on the stand. The coffin was still there as I climbed into the pulpit to read. My mum had never lain still for so long. She'd be hurrying me along up those pulpit steps if she could. 'Come on, get a move on, we haven't got forever,' she'd say. She has eternity now. I saw a sea of familiar faces, including David right at the back with an unusual heaviness on his face. There were waves of tears across the room, emotion crashing toward me as I carefully opened an oversized Bible to somewhere in the middle. The Bible was nearly as heavy as the coffin. If only Kindle had existed back then, I could have done the reading one-handed.

Words from Psalm 139 spilled from my lips, the irony making me choke: 'Even darkness will not be dark to you; the night will shine like the day… for you knit me together in my mother's womb. I praise you because I am fearfully and wonderfully made.' Yes, the body that carried my twin sister and me and my older brother into the world, the womb which nurtured and protected us, which made us wonderfully, was now lifeless in a box. Just down there. Stuck, fearlessly stuck. This is the deal. We all get a start line and a finish line. But life isn't like flat-pack furniture, we have to work out the bit that joins the two lines without an Allen key and cartoon instructions.

In the cemetery the sun tried to peek through greyness. The box was lowered into a cold hole where the fingers of the sun would never reach. Where was my mum now? She was bones, she was earth, she was air. Free to fly to wherever she chose. More power than Icarus, more strength in her wings than feathers and wax, she could touch the sun.

I stayed strong for as long as I could at the wake afterwards. Welcoming guests, handing out vol-au-vents and nodding after people said things to me. I spoke with Uncle Andrew and his family, but I don't recall a word that was said. I was already retreating, like a tide turning and fleeing for some distant shore.

That night at home, I collapsed onto the sofa. All I heard was sobbing, my sobbing. All I saw was a blurred ceiling. During those hours something was taken from me, like a reservoir evaporating to the sky. Drained, I couldn't physically move. My wife fetched a duvet, placed it over me, stroked my face, and let me sob until from exhaustion I slept.

Is the process of loss a straight line from A to B? No, it looks more like a 2-year-old's scribbled drawing, lines going off the edges of the page at every chance.

I threw the television remote control across the lounge when it didn't work immediately; I kicked my son's empty cot when trying to lower the mattress; I thumped the walls of my kitchen with my fists and headbutted the floor. As if the floor would open up.

'What does anything matter?' I said. Death had turned me into the philosopher's apprentice. There weren't any Stages of Grief. No tick-box list to go through or map to say You Are Here.

I stared at the sun and wondered how many more times I would see it; calculating my mum lived for 21,217 days. I figured some were DAYS! but most were probably just d... a... y... s. I wondered about my own life. Why did so many days seem to be written in font size 6, not font size 76? I wanted Noticeable not Invisible. Fulfilling not Forgotten. I didn't want to slip away under a duvet. You don't get over grief, you just inch towards being reconciled to a permanent hole that now exists. 'Are we nearly there yet?' we ask. No. There isn't a destination. You just keep going.

It was difficult adjusting to Mum not being there. For several years it was like our family had a puncture, losing momentum and balance now she was gone, as well as the roast dinners and the endings to all those unfinished stories.

Getting my feet out of bed and onto the carpet seemed like an accomplishment.

'Look, I'm still here!' But nobody said 'well done' for getting out of bed. No gold stars for daring to open the curtains.

'Depression is 100,000 abusive voices, as if the Devil has Tourette's,' says Ruby Wax. If only we could unscrew our heads some days. But we're not Lego people. The mind, body and soul are fused together. Is depression the same as grief? You're too absorbed by what you don't have than what you do. It's all Absence. My wife was so patient, waiting for me to return, keeping our family ticking along.

People speak to you but all you see is their mouth opening and closing. You hear nothing because your mental Wi-Fi has lost its signal. Grief draws a heavily lined curtain between you and the world and makes you randomly and suddenly think about lilac duvets, disposable pants and creaking stairs, trying to rewind the movie of those last few days, re-edit the episode and desperately change something. But death isn't compatible with Photoshop. The past is Saved and Filed, never Deleted.

Grief proved a bigger experience than I expected. I behaved as if it was linear, a single line drawn down the family tree: Mum and Me. What about the other dimensions? My dad losing his wife. My brother and sister losing their mum too. My son losing his grandma. My wife losing her 'new mum'. My grandparents losing their daughter. They had been too frail to travel 4 hours from Wales for her funeral so they had watched a video recording of it. They could rewind and fast-forward and pause and mute their daughter's funeral. But they couldn't be there.

Loss can feel enormous. You feel lost. Automatic doesn't work anymore. You open your eyes and everything looks different.

The first time I dreamt about my mum after her death was 4 months later, in November. I was free of the numbness that follows death, and I was, although I didn't recognise it then, at the nadir of my grief.

And then the dream. The simplest dream, where I was lying in bed when my mum came to my bedside, like when I was a child. She stroked my head. As I slept, I felt the weight of her hand, the press of her fingers on my scalp, the slow movement from the top of my head to the base of my neck. I sensed her smile, letting her say goodbye. Letting her say to me this time, 'Sleep well, my beautiful.' When I awoke, something in me had changed.

Something stirred, a desire to ask new questions, a search for new things. A quest to find out what I was made of before being stuck in a box and lowered into the guts of the earth.

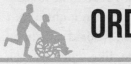

ORDINARY MAGIC

*The oak fought the wind and was broken, the
willow bent when it must and survived.*

Robert Jordan

Some people arrive in your life for a limited time. They bring a
message you need to know, or an opportunity you need to grasp.
They don't show up with a flashing neon sign, or a fanfare of
trumpets. Usually they just slip into your life quietly, so you can't
quite put your finger on when they started to affect the trajectory
of your life. But by the time they leave they have put down roots.
Alchemy has taken place. You can never be the same.

It was my friend David who was the listening ear through my
months of grief. During the 7 months before my mum's death
and the 7 months after, three of my grandparents also died,
including one on Christmas Eve 2005, and one on our son's first
birthday in February 2006. David took me out for spaghetti
carbonara and allowed my story to unravel incoherently like
the pasta twirled on my fork.

'You don't have to work it all out,' he said, 'things won't stay as they are.'

David was taller and thinner than most people you meet. You could feel his voice under your feet, a voice that reverberated through you like the engine of a sports car. I met him when I was 22, and loved hanging out with him even though he was three decades older and I got neck ache talking with him. He just did everything differently. Thought about everything differently. He was like jazz in a world swamped by shopping-mall music.

He was also the busiest man I ever met – looking after businesses in fashion and technology, a consultant travelling to and fro across the Atlantic, taking care of his vineyard in the heart of England, and being a husband and father of four. David made too many promises to help others than he could ever keep. He wanted to give life everything he had. His life was loaded up like a long-distance train in India, with no space left in it, or on it, but he knew where he wanted to go even when he seemed to go off the tracks. He loved going off the tracks. He needed three lives. The one he had certainly wasn't long enough.

One evening, early in 2006, I went to visit him in Warwick Hospital during the latter stages of his treatment for bladder cancer. I parked in the hospital car park and approached the automatic doors to the building, the glass smeared with hand marks as though people were trying to escape. The door hesitated to open, sussing me out, wondering for whom the flowers I was holding were intended. The door slid back. I strode down the corridor, taking big strides. I followed the signs to the ward where he was recovering. Surely this place is just a temporary pit stop, I thought. David didn't belong here.

He sat upright in bed to meet me, as if my appearance had been like lightning, and looked at the bunch of white roses I was holding, wrapped in plastic. He smiled.

'How are you, Chris?' he asked. Every question carried weight. David had this way of paying attention to you, as if you were the only person in the room. Yet I knew him well enough to know that he probably had a hundred loose ends in his head to deal with.

I pulled up a chair to his bedside, scraping the floor with the metal legs. The faded hospital gown hung off his shoulders like it didn't want to be there. A tub of grapes rested on his tray, and a travel clock ticked, snatching each moment away. The other patients appeared out for the count, as if on Pause. Their lives drained, bottled, labelled, shelved. Not so with David.

'How do you cope?' I asked, and handed him the roses.

Just four words. But I guess I was also asking: Why is this happening to you? Are you leaving soon? Why haven't I made more of our time together? Are the roses OK?

He chuckled. A smile formed beneath the bags under his eyes. One simple laugh revealing the immensity of the man, laughing in the face of death.

'I think about everything I'm thankful for,' he said. As if it was obvious. He hadn't practised a response or peeked at the back of the book for the Right Answer. David had this way of taking stock, weighing it all up, and coming up with a conclusion nobody else had considered.

He looked up at the ceiling tiles, then continued. 'Being content in all circumstances. What other option do I have?' and leaned over to arrange the roses, which looked sparse in the vase. I could think of alternatives to contentment.

Since the hospital visit with the white roses, and David's laughing, the question 'how do you cope?' has become a fascination to me. So much of our lives hinges on our capacity to cope from moment to moment and month to month, and the mindset we carry in the face of difficulty. What do we pay attention to when trouble seems to overwhelm us? I wasn't a runner then. If I was, I'd have had an answer to my question.

What David modelled to me can be distilled into a single word: resilience. By that, I mean the ability to become psychologically stronger and healthier, within reason, after something bad happens. Facing adversity head-on, not hiding behind the sofa. It's the capacity to handle uncertainty without becoming a control freak. Showing gratitude for what you do have, not complaining about what you don't. Resilience says we can do well, even when life isn't how we thought it would be. After all, we can't escape trouble any more than climb out of our skin. Difficulties get our attention, like a bucket of ice-cold water over the head, waking us up to reality. And they offer a quiet invitation, whispering: What do you want to make of me? Shake an angry fist at the sky, or lift your head and face it? Whichever attitude you go for, heads or tails, determines everything that follows.

Professor Ann Masten, a child psychologist from the University of Minnesota has a term for all this: 'Ordinary Magic,' she says. I like that. I think David would too.

'Ordinary Magic is about doing OK despite difficulties in the past or present,' she says. This doesn't mean we pretend all is fine. That would be dishonest and dangerous, but we can take care in how we interpret what happens to us and around us. We always have a choice, even if it takes a moment to look up at the ceiling and notice it. The choice that is, not the ceiling. Resilience is hard-wired, available to us all. It's when we encounter difficulties that our Ordinary Magic appears, not in a mask, cape and brightly coloured tights, but in our thoughts, intentions and actions. A resilient mindset is like an old photograph; it needs the dark to develop, to reveal the wonder hiding inside.

David changed my paradigm of myself. Instead of thinking there was something wrong with me, that I was somehow deficient or in need of fixing (a legacy from school days, I suspect), he gave me a new lens to look through, one about inside strength: What was I really capable of? How could I play my part fully in the world? Because if I don't live my life fully, the world won't get it from elsewhere.

'You're more than you think you are,' he used to say, and the words would loiter in my mind as I tried to untangle their knot of wisdom. It was an inverted way of perceiving life, which didn't come naturally to me. Optimism was his realism. He and scout-leader Skip would have liked each other. They'd have spent nights just looking up, drinking David's wine, pointing to new possibilities with their long arms, a fuzzy patch of stars no doubt winking back at them with pleasure.

David couldn't see the stars from his hospital bed, but he was born for the outdoors. He often got me working alongside him, involving me in his life, whether in his vineyard, garden or out on the road delivering training talks around the country. Perhaps I was just cheap labour.

'Your biggest room for improvement is in your strengths,' he would say, as we pruned vines in his vineyard together. And as I dropped gnarled branches to the earth, a mounting pile of broken tangled twigs at my feet, new ideas surged with energy within me. One of those was to start a mentoring initiative for young people to help reduce their distress, build resilience and inspire possibility. David agreed there was a need but dismantled my idea into tiny parts, not convinced it would ever get the funding it needed.

But the idea became so compelling I left my three part-time jobs – one teaching, one as a youth worker and one gardening – and, with help from friends, I went all out to get it going. David had installed a belief that I was capable of more than I thought, and it ran deeper than any of his well-argued doubts and his rare bout of scepticism. The mentoring charity I established, called Lifespace Trust, has just celebrated 10 years of existence, and has mentored over a thousand young people through a team of trained mentors, mostly volunteers. The work keeps growing. David would be proud of me, probably. He'd also say something to keep me restless and on the edge of annoyance.

He used to wear a T-shirt with the slogan: 'If it ain't growing, it ain't living.' For David, nothing was fixed, not capability nor talent. Life moved with a relentless rhythm.

'Once our minds are stretched by a new idea,' said American physician and poet Oliver Wendell-Holmes, 'they can never return to their original dimension.' David definitely stretched my mind. To be fair, sometimes he totally did my head in.

Today in our back garden we have a white rose bush. It reminds me of my hospital visit to David and my question about coping. His laugh and cursory glance at the ceiling and attitude of Doing OK in life, despite difficulties. Being thankful despite struggle. The roses have such a sweet smell, I always reach my nose in for more. They don't hold back. Like David, they offer everything they have.

When I pluck the pears each autumn from the tree in my garden, and bite into their flesh, I remember each pear has known the glaring sun, the abandonment of the night and the violence of the wind. I cannot remove any of this from within the pear. The pear has been in the elements and the elements are in the pear. Each live within the other. David helped me accept that life is like this. Within faith exists doubt. Within love we touch loss. Within struggle hides resilience. We cannot have one without being in reach of the other.

What was the message he infused into my life? Lift up your head. Point your life towards the horizon. Whatever you do, don't get stuck. David introduced me to Ordinary Magic, and my uncle gave me the encouragement and example to express it through running. We are a family in need of each other. It was the perfect recipe to fall in love with marathons.

WE ALL HAVE TO START SOMEWHERE

Start with the end in mind.

Stephen R. Covey

I don't know exactly when I became a Runner, but I know why and how.

At first my newfound pursuit was about running away from death. Then slowly, with each unrhythmic mile, I started running back towards life.

For 8 months after my mum's death grief tangled my headspace. I felt like a magnet for sad news.

'Sorry, wrong address,' I wanted to say, 'please return to sender', with a thick line through my name. Every day started with confusion, like my centre of gravity had been stolen. The family tree had been turned upside down, the names at the top now in the ground. It's as if all I knew and loved had gone into those coffins, lost deep into the earth, or incinerated by flames.

Then came my birthday in March. I needed to make an effort. I picked up the razor and shaved, hardly recognising the man staring back at me. Or staring through me, I couldn't tell. His cheeks were chubbier. Eyes sullen. Perhaps the real me had gone up in flames too.

'Where shall we go?' my wife asked.

'Anywhere but here,' I said, as I put on my scarf and gloves.

We drove to a National Trust garden in neighbouring Gloucestershire. My wife clasped my hand as we walked through the patchwork of gardens at Hidcote Manor, past the battalions of tulips, standing erect, so many closed flower heads, as if keeping their thoughts to themselves. How long would it be until they spilled their colours, lighting up the garden like fireworks?

We stopped for coffee in the outdoor courtyard. A blackbird stood nearby, a sentinel warbling its familiar jingle. Perhaps it was excited about spring. Getting outdoors helped, my strength began to return, a surge of life back through the earth started to recharge me.

'I think I can move on from the loss of my mum,' I said. 'I'm going to draw a line under my grief.' It felt good to say it like that, a decision on my birthday, because 8 months of grief since her death was quite enough.

Thirteen days later the phone rang at 7 a.m. You never get good news at 7 a.m. It was David's wife, Meryl.

'David's died,' she said. I stood in my kitchen holding a spoon for breakfast in one hand and the phone in the other. Perhaps the spoon helped me keep balance. There were no silly euphemisms, only the honest fact, her voice flushed with peacefulness. I'd had nearly 2 weeks of being free of grief. A chance to clear my throat. And now my best friend was dead.

The morning of Meryl's phone call I walked a mile and a half to my office in Stratford-upon-Avon. Everything seemed normal, as if nothing had moved. The traffic queues were all present and correct, van drivers tapped steering wheels, getting as close as possible to the car in front. But everything is always changing. I walked up the stairs into my windowless office, slumped in my chair and thought about how I would not see my best friend again, not on this earth. I pulled out a notepad and wrote a list of all the people I needed to telephone to tell them of David's death, having promised Meryl I would.

For the next 5 hours I sat in my chair and made those calls. 'I'm calling to let you know David died this morning.' No matter how many times I said it, it felt like the first time to a new receiver of the news. Sometimes the call lasted 2 minutes, the other person being quiet, finding enough strength just to blink and say 'thank you' for telling them. Other times the call lasted half an hour and I shifted from news giver to listener, as friends of David relayed their anecdotes and were 'so sorry' for the news. Sometimes the emotion caught in my voice and I had to take a moment to compose myself before picking up the phone again, dialling the next number on the list. And the next number. So many numbers, just one story, ticking each off as I got through.

After each call came the silence, like after turning the radio off. I considered those hours amongst the most privileged and exhausting of my life, but I think David would be relieved I didn't do it through Facebook.

When David's cremation took place in early April, it was in the same room where I once led a cremation service for an elderly lady. Everything had gone well, until I had to press the button under the lectern for the coffin to begin its slow exit and the curtains to wrap around the small stage, like the end of a theatre performance. All timed perfectly with a piece of organ music. The staff at the crematorium told me beforehand that under no circumstances must I press the button twice. The room was silent. Music began. There were tears from family and friends as I pressed the button and the coffin started to move. But then it got stuck; the curtains froze in terror, clanking to a halt. The organ continued, oblivious, as everyone twitched their heads, from the coffin to me back to the coffin, wondering what on earth I'd done. The music finished. Everyone looked confused as the coffin refused to budge. There was only one thing for it. I hit that button as hard as I could, and in the awkward post-music hush, the coffin squeaked away reluctantly and the curtains slid themselves shut in a sulk.

'I heard how hard you hit that button. It ain't ever gonna work again,' a relative of the deceased said to me afterwards.

David's coffin didn't do a disappearing act either, but it was deliberate, not a malfunction. Instead, Meryl walked across the room full of wooden seats, knotted with sadness, right up to the raised platform, the tap-tap of her heels echoing on the floor. Then she rested a card on top of the coffin which read 'End of Part One'.

Part Two of David's funeral was held later in the day in the hay barn next to his home and vineyard. With everyone sat either on chairs or hay bales, I told the story of a day out together in Cambridge when he drove me in his Lotus Elise, roof down all the way, enjoying September sunshine. It was one of the best days of my life, soaking in his company and friendship, and taking the time to look up, literally and metaphorically. It was also the day of a national fuel crisis. We walked to Pembroke College Chapel, where he and Meryl got married, and gazed up at the ceiling, which was harder for me being so short. We listened to a performance of Messiaens on the cello, each note vibrating its way through me. We watched a film and went to a seminar at the university. Then we went to return home, but his fuel gauge was in red so he pulled onto a petrol station forecourt, one car lost amongst a hundred, like refugee hands at the back of an aid lorry. We waited. His face turned towards mine.

'Are you OK with taking a risk?' he said. He smiled, reversed out of the queue, leaving a snake of vehicles in front and behind and we hit the open road, not knowing if we would make it back home. David looked at a crisis as an opportunity in disguise. Perhaps he was trying to tell me: 'You've got more in the tank than you think you have.' We made it home.

An image from David's funeral stays with me. It's how I best remember him: David standing in his vineyard, pouring a glass of his own homegrown red wine, sun shining, him smiling, content in that circumstance.

There is a time to mourn, for grief has much to teach us. We only grieve if we have loved. But it can hang around too long and cause us to get stuck in our lives, becoming a destination. Life is not a permanent fixture; I wanted to get a move on, like my mum always told me to.

'All our sorrows can be borne if we can put them into a story,' said author Isak Dinesen. We start to change when we change the story we tell.

After the cremation I decided I needed to wrestle my life back from the grasping hands of grief. To tell a different story. I needed to find a way of pouring my heart out, like David with his wine. I couldn't get stuck here, death as my life partner. How could I draw the curtains on my grief to a close?

'When we change the way we look at our sufferings, we can go in search of wonders despite the pain,' said psychologist Boris Cyrulnik. So I hit the button on my life as hard as I could and started running, not knowing what it would lead to.

Thinking back, running was my escape during my uncomfortable grey-socked days at school. I didn't know about being strong in the classroom, but I found some inside strength on the cross-country course with Mr Pegden, my P.E. teacher. All the kids liked him, and his squint gave him a sense of vulnerability. He would lean against a chestnut tree, chewing gum, as we got into our stride doing three laps of the playing fields. I surprised myself by running well. I remember on one occasion actually being scared my legs were going to fall off, as I overtook classmate after classmate to finish as one of the first few boys. Running became my refuge away from the teasing and name-calling, inevitable given I was short with a bad haircut. The cross-country course seemed the only place I wasn't restricted by the elastic on my trousers. Mr Pegden would give me short words of encouragement. 'Well done, Spriggsy.' 'Good running, Sprigglet.' He was keeping an eye on me, I'm just not sure which one.

Fast-forward 26 years, and firmly off Mr Pegden's radar, I decided to emulate my uncle and join 38,000 others in the London Marathon. It would be my first. I had a year to make my physical training shift the weight of my emotional cargo. I wanted to find out if I could run further than I'd gone before.

My first run was in a cotton T-shirt, 10-year-old trainers and my wife's jogging bottoms. I started running in the dark, but so would you if you had women's jogging bottoms on.

I was only 100 metres into the run, when I heard shouting. I realised it was me: 'Come on then! COME ON!' Pumping my fists in the air, like a zealous aerobics instructor, I was having an argument with the sky, or my pent-up grief perhaps. Was this me flexing my muscle, hoping to become something I wasn't? I wanted to face up to the subtle voice in my head that was telling me to go back home, so I told it to shut up. Grief must not become a full stop. I began running to find the start of something, to escape my depression as well as catch up with the world. Two-for-the-price-of-one. The physical movement helped unravel the mess in my mind, thread by thread. I managed to complete my first run, clocking 2.5 miles to kick-start my running career.

From May to October, in the immediate months after David's death, my weekly mileage was irregular, never quite breaking double figures. I started running four or five times each week. My plan included the happy trinity of marathon training: a fast run plus a hilly run plus a long run. After a few weeks the training plan started to look like a Sudoku puzzle without an answer.

My long run each weekend went from 1 mile in May to 3 miles in August, to 7 miles in October. That was the aim, an hour of running by October. It was a slow process and progress came in tiny steps. Are there rules to running? Yes, but rules which work in the classroom don't work on the road. You have to make up your own, and copy those of others wherever that works. Nobody's marking your ability to run. When I started training I didn't know about fast and slow twitch muscle fibres, or the difference between a tempo run (maintaining good pace throughout) and a progression run (getting gradually faster each mile). I hadn't heard about eating within half an hour after a run to maximise the body's replacement of glycogen (the substance that muscles use to store energy after that energy has been broken down from carbohydrates). To me glycogen sounded like something you put in rockets. There were so many things I didn't know, but if we waited to know everything, when would we ever start anything? Every writer went through a time of not knowing the alphabet. Every athlete spent time crawling on their knees. I was a work in progress. What I had going for me was knowing my Why. My Reason. You can get a long way when you know your reason.

In the autumn I returned from my first run of an hour, simultaneously delighted and demoralised. Outdoors the loss stopped strangling me, I breathed more easily and noticed things. Simple things like blackberries ripening, and how they hung in tightly knit families from roadside bushes. The sort of thing I missed hurtling by in a car. Slowly discipline took shape. It felt fantastic to have clocked over 60 minutes of running for the first time in my life, kicking conkers and listening to honking geese above, migrating their way south in an orderly queue like they knew where they were going (which, of course, they always do). But the thought of repeating this distance more than four times over in a marathon was daunting. It was easy to forget how far I had come.

I decided to aim for a 4-hour finish time, even though I hadn't yet heard if I had a place in the race. That was the unexplained holy grail for marathon-finishing times. I did the sums, an average pace of 9 minutes 9 seconds per mile, for every mile.

As my weekend long runs climbed into double figures, I started getting emails from my uncle. He speckled his emails with advice: 'Enter a local race so you know what it's like running with others at speed.' 'Better to arrive on the start line a little under-prepared than over-trained.' He stretched my intentions: 'Make sure you do at least one twenty-miler. Twenty miles is halfway, you know!' I didn't correct his maths because he was hinting at something more psychological. 'Make sure you get decent trainers and get your running gait properly analysed.' I made notes of it all. I created a folder on my computer called 'Running', which was short for 'Uncle Andrew's No-Hype Guide to Marathon Training'.

At the start of December the London Marathon race-ballot results were announced. I'd been telling everyone I was definitely doing it, nodding my head when I talked about it, but the first thing I saw on the cover of my copy of *Marathon News* magazine resting on the doormat was 'SORRY'. Something must be wrong, surely? Successful ballot entrants got the same magazine but with 'CONGRATULATIONS' across the cover. I realised I didn't have a place in the World's Greatest Race. This shouldn't have been such a big surprise, given the ratio is one place for every eight requests, but didn't they know how far I'd come? How many cowpats I'd stepped in on my cross-country route? The times I'd thrown my voice to the clouds? How uncomfortable my wife's jogging bottoms were that first day?

I felt deflated. I stomped my feet. My inner 7-year-old resurfaced. Then my sister-in-law Ruth emailed and suggested I run for a charity. Despite the magazine being abundant with 'run for charity' adverts, the idea hadn't been on my radar. Sometimes I'm oblivious to the obvious.

I applied for a place with Cancer Research UK but was refused. I sulked again, before trying Macmillan Cancer

Support, who had provided nursing care to my mum, so I knew first-hand the cause was a worthwhile one.

Several days later I was at work in a school, sat in a room the size of a broom cupboard, waiting for a young person to turn up for their mentoring session. My phone vibrated in my pocket, with news bursting to get out. A young voice spoke, a lady from Macmillan Cancer Support saying I'd secured a Golden Bond London Marathon race place with them, with a conditional fundraising target of £1,800.

'Are you sure?' I asked her. 'Why have you picked me?' She laughed at my questions.

'You have a story to tell,' she said, 'we know this matters to you.'

C. S. Lewis had his wardrobe into the world of Narnia; J. K. Rowling had her platform 9¾ into the world of Hogwarts; I had my broom cupboard into a world of New Beginnings. I sprinted on the spot, pumped my arms, and squealed with joy. Then I realised a teacher was watching me from across the foyer through the reinforced glass window, shaking her head. I imagined a tut-tut from her lips.

But I was IN THE RACE and no reinforced glass could hold me back.

I felt ready to take on and beat the English winter. I turned off the alarm at 6 a.m. and put on my running kit in the pitch black of the bedroom, as if preparing to go on a bank raid. I felt reloaded, ready for the icy pavements before dawn opened its eyes. Running was my version of making a rude and inappropriate gesture at death, with two feet instead of two fingers. The darkness would not overcome me.

The twilight mornings of strategic tiptoeing to avoid creaky floorboards and get out for a run without waking anyone were tough on my wife, who was pregnant, due with our second child in late January. She'd already battled against several months of pre-natal depression.

The plan was to have the baby at home, in a birthing pool purchased for the occasion. The day after the due date, her contractions started. Brilliant, a 'Monday's child, fair of face'. It took 3 hours for me to fill the birthing pool as none of the hoses fitted the house taps. I shuffled between lounge and kitchen, pans of boiling water in each hand like a competitor on *It's A Knockout*, spilling it over the floor. My back ached like crazy, but I decided not to tell my wife who was lying on the sofa having contractions.

Her contractions receded. A false alarm. Twenty-four hours passed. I waited at work for news, but nothing. Finally at 3 a.m. on the Wednesday everything kicked back in. Progress was quick. Only one of the community midwives arrived in time. The baby's head appeared, dark hair. Hannah puffed. Gas. Air. Gas. Air. Expletive. A baby entered life in the water and was thrust onto my wife's chest; they were connected in every way. Air hit the receptors on her skin, triggering her first ever oxygen-loaded breaths. It was a girl, a beautiful girl, with a look of shock on her face. She became ours. With the umbilical cord clamped, I cut through the feeding pipe that joined mother and child. There was resistance as I cut the cord, like I was setting them free.

'Her name,' I said, with pride and wonder in my voice, 'is Maisie-Joy Beatrice.' It means 'Pearl of Joy, Bringer of Happiness'. A name chosen with our story in mind. My mother-in-law, a midwife herself and up from Essex especially for the birth, handed round cups of tea and cupcakes, carefully stepping around my water spillages and the suitcases of medical equipment. As my wife held our daughter I stepped outdoors. The 4 a.m. midwinter chill slapped my face. I looked into the darkness, and imagined the stars striking up like an orchestra, humming and singing with pleasure. I stared at them, burning globes, as bright as on any other night I'd looked.

'Sorrow may last for a night-time, but joy comes in the morning,' wrote a poet centuries ago. It was a turning point, 9 months in the making.

Our first day with Maisie-Joy was full of arranging flowers, washing white linen and, in those moments when we stopped, letting our fingers trace her wrinkled skin as if drawing invisible maps upon her, signatures of love. I was secretly marking out new running routes on her.

On Thursday morning, with almost no sleep in 3 days, I ran, no longer beating the pavement into submission with grief, but running as if I had feathers in my feet, inhaling morning air like I was the one who was newborn, sunlight seeping into my skin. Bare trees waved like cheerleaders, and the earth seemed to laugh beneath me. My feet and the earth were in love again. Everything was new as I ran, life forever changed, each step was joy, Joy, JOY. The 2007 London Marathon beckoned, and each run took me closer. I was sure all that carrying water to the birth pool had developed my core strength.

Seven weeks before the marathon I took my uncle's advice and got my running gait checked out at a running shop. I would have described my running style as 'happy', but I suspected they would provide a more technical description. I had mentioned to a friend about the decrepit state of my trainers, which had after all lasted a decade.

'They've got me this far,' I said. A few days later he sent me a cheque for £120 for a new pair.

I visited the 'Up and Running' shop in Cheltenham, nearly an hour's drive away but the closest place I could have my running gait analysed by video. Watching yourself run in slow motion on playback is an odd experience; really they should play the *Chariots of Fire* theme tune.

'Your pronation is quite pronounced,' the manager summarised. Afterwards I sat on a cushioned stool in the middle of the shop, conspicuous and clueless, as he explained pronation – inward rolling feet. He disappeared to the back of the shop and returned carrying a stack of shoeboxes. I didn't know how to say the brand names – Saucony (Sork-A-Nee) from my lips became 'Sauce-Oh-Nee'. In the end I went for a pair of Brooks Adrenaline GTS, which sounded like a sports car, but I could pronounce Brooks, and the shop manager let me put them on and go for a run around town. I'd never had so much 'cushioning'; the trainers were like a sports bra for my feet. My Brooks worked like mini pogo sticks. The general advice is that a pair of trainers should last up to 500 running miles, but mine last for over 1,000 each year, with almost no injuries. Mixing up road running with trails probably helps.

At home I checked in my 'Running' folder on the computer. What other advice from my uncle did I need to follow? 'Make sure you have a practice race so you get used to running with others at speed,' he had said. I researched what was around in March that would give my legs a stretch and test my stamina.

I turned up for a rural 15-mile race in Banbury in Oxfordshire, my first race since school sports day half a lifetime ago. I stood toward the rear of the pack, in a faded cotton T-shirt and spanking new trainers. I ate a banana as quickly as I could, so it bulged in both cheeks, and regretted this for the next hour, but I finished the race with gritted teeth and bits of banana between them. Later that day my uncle emailed me, having looked up the results online. Apparently 1 hour 54 minutes was 'good going'.

I didn't know then about stretching your legs afterwards, or peanut butter on toast as the perfect protein-recovery snack. I wasn't clued up on getting antioxidants into my system (anything with vitamins A, C or E) to neutralise the harmful effects of free radicals created by exercise. I didn't know not to wear cotton, which became very uncomfortable once soaked in sweat. All that knowledge was still in the future pipeline, but the idea of finishing my first marathon in 4 hours seemed in reaching distance.

I started whispering 'You can do this, son' to myself in the mirror. I had no idea why I addressed myself as 'son'.

Running is rarely an injury-free journey. Grape-sized blisters, black toenails, light-headedness from mineral depletion, nausea, lactate acid in the knees, a stiff neck, aching shoulders, tight hamstrings, tender calf muscles, a dry throat, a dodgy tummy and rushed visits to the toilet (or hedge), plus headaches from dehydration. You'd be very unlucky to get all that in one go, mind you. There is purpose to discomfort, a correlation between effort and enjoyment, and most ailments have a simple remedy if you read up on them or ask around. The right-sized shoes, swapping tarmac for trails, a sensible pace and plan for your ability, and being hydrated before you go out will conquer many problems. Not all, but many. One thing I would never do again is have off-the-shelf orthotics, which turned a minor foot strain into a 6-week lay-off.

Having rest days also works wonders, giving your body time to recuperate and integrate the training. I followed my plan meticulously. Some evenings I just stood and stared at all the ticks on my chart just for the dopamine rush.

In the week before Marathon Day I created an acronym, 'CRASH', to help me focus. It stands for:

Carb up – eat plenty of rice, toast and sweet potatoes to top up the body's glycogen stores in the 3 days before the race.

Rest well – aim for an extra hour of sleep each night in the week before the race, as you may not sleep well the night immediately before, and it's while you sleep that the immune system switches from 'defend' mode to 'repair' mode.

Analyse the route – look at the map and check travel arrangements, baggage drop, running terrain and elevation, water stations and provisions, etc.

Strategise – think about your target running pace, equal pace being the most efficient if you want to achieve a certain time; have a nutrition strategy for before, during and after the race; check your equipment, consulting the weather forecast to decide on running kit and whether you'll need to wear a bin liner at the start to keep you warm; stock up on energy supplies.

Hydrate – make sure your pee is pale-straw colour or lighter to know you're hydrated.

One morning, just days before the race, I picked up my razor and looked at the man in the bathroom mirror. He had changed. The chubby cheeks had gone. The grief was falling away, like leaves from trees. Stripped but ready. The man, he seemed, he seemed... present again.

* * *

I went to the London Marathon Expo (the pre-race exhibition) at London's ExCeL Centre on the Friday, something that only comes with the really big races. Everyone was flapping programmes at their faces. April felt like July. We were 5 weeks into a spring heatwave and the forecast was 22 degrees for race day. On the Saturday night I went into a restaurant in the heart of London for the Macmillan Cancer Support pre-race pasta party, which got me fired up after the motivational talk from a double-amputee runner showing off his 'running blades'. It was good to meet some of the other 800 Macmillan runners and swap stories. I was delighted to have raised over £4,500 for the charity in my first sponsorship attempt, a testimony to how loved my mum and David were, as well as respect for the cause. Now my legs just had to deliver a stack of miles.

I arrived with my family at my mother-in-law's house in Chadwell Heath, on the edge of east London. It was less than 12 hours until the race started and I was too excited to sleep. I stood on her doorstep and looked up at the night sky. Our daughter was not quite 3 months old, but the night reminded me of the one on which she was born. It was much warmer, but those stars were still humming with joy. My legs were ready to run through the city, and leave the footsteps of my sadness behind me, for a tide of runners behind to erase forever. About an hour's drive away, my uncle was laying out his running kit, Vaseline, safety pins and trainers, ready to run the London Marathon for the twelfth time. It was the first time we would run in the same race.

I didn't know exactly when I became a Runner, but I liked where it was taking me.

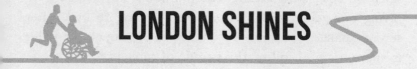

LONDON SHINES

*You only ever grow as a human being if
you're outside your comfort zone.*

Percy Cerutty

I go to sleep after one a.m. My alarm sounds at 5.40 a.m. I tiptoe downstairs, eat some toast in a daydream, then drink coffee. 'Nothing unusual for race day,' my uncle has told me.

I've kept the same routine for every marathon since. Item by item, I pick up my running kit, laid out the night before with precision, like a crime scene. Race preparation verges on obsessive compulsive disorder, nothing is left to chance, nothing random. Safety pins are triple-checked. Through narrow eyes I wipe Vaseline between my toes. I lace up my trainers as if preparing for execution. I double-check my number: 41077. Today, I AM that number. I take a minute to close the front door so as not to wake my family. It's such a clean sky for April, like a new start. At Chadwell Heath train station I spy on other runners to see how they've attached their timing chip to their trainers. My mind has so many questions: When should I consume my energy gels? Does my bumbag look silly? Where are the toilets? Did I put enough Vaseline on my nipples? Not things I usually think of first thing in the morning.

Station by station the carriage fills with runners and the smell of Deep Heat cream. The journey is not helped by a raving evangelist telling us we are all going to hell. After several changes (of train, not underwear, although the latter is appropriate), I follow the parade of runners off the train, swarming under the insistent sun towards the 'Red Start' in Greenwich Park, marching like football fans towards a stadium, focused, hopeful. Perhaps we are going to hell sooner than we think. I enter the park and decide to walk round shaking people's hands, 'Great job!' I say. They look confused, but I think getting to the start line is an achievement in itself. Unfortunately, some have just come out from the Portaloos, and they look concerned about what I've just said to them.

I squeeze through the railings into my allotted sub-4-hour race pen, like a sheep on market day, then sit in the pen clutching my knees. There's half an hour until the start, my backside goes numb. Waiting, just waiting. Somewhere a few hundred metres away in Blackheath, my uncle Andrew waits on a different start line, the 'Blue Start', for the same race. The London Marathon is possibly the only race in the world with three separate start lines and one finish line.

The build-up is something you never forget, your legs aching with anticipation and glycogen from triple helpings of pasta the night before, wondering whether you can run 26.2 miles. Or not. Knowing only time will tell. There's no boredom here, just the hope of glory and the promise of pain.

I see the BBC film crew on the scaffold tower beyond the gates to Greenwich Park, getting that iconic panoramic shot of all the runners congested and eager, a temporary congregation waiting to be poured out like a sacrifice onto the city streets.

My uncle and I count ourselves part of one of the biggest clubs in the world, full of people with different world views and outlooks, but who share a love for putting one foot in front of the other. Running isn't just a behaviour, a leisure pursuit or a hobby. It's more than that. Running is about belonging to a bigger story of overcoming. This enormous diverse community embraces the physically overweight; recovering addicts; youngsters half our age who run twice as fast; pensioners who felt they had (metaphorically) missed the bus; mums stressed out by kids; dads stressed out by wives who are stressed out by kids. Runners are one massive dysfunctional family, many of whom love chasing personal-best times (or PBs, in running parlance), tongues hanging out by their ankles at finish lines. People who by day have respectable jobs, but by evening metamorphose into running-stat nerds, drooling over course profiles, split mile times, calorie intake and training plans with more intervals than the entire collection of West End theatres. Runners love becoming their best versions of themselves. In search of more. More to find and more to give.

To one side of me is a lad who turned 18 years old yesterday, likely to be the youngest of today's 38,000 runners. On the other side is Bill, in his sixties, who sprained his ankle yesterday whilst walking his dog. Yesterday was a big day for the pair of them. We sit together, talking, other runners bouncing up and down around us.

Unlike my uncle in his twelfth London Marathon outing, I don't have a clue what to expect or what I'm capable of. You suspect you're connecting to something so much bigger than yourself, as the BBC cameraman does his best to capture it all. The start line is an overloading experience for the senses. The magic of the marathon can never be squeezed back into the genie's lamp.

I listen to the sounds: the purring helicopter with a camera crew eyeing us like wildebeest on the savannah; the nervous chatter and laughter of runners; then whooping cheers as we take our first tentative steps; hooters and whistles blaring at the roadside; thousands of feet, in padded cocoons, slap-slapping the road; the sound of high-fives and clap-clapping with kids on the pavement, and your name being called out (it's important to remember to somehow display your name on your vest for this very reason). The sound is all around from the start to the end. A festival of noise.

Then there are the smells. The wafts of Deep Heat on legs reach your nostrils, and the abrupt pong of cleaning chemicals pours out from the parade of portable toilets in the park; later, there's the tangy odour of orange drinks for mile upon mile as you persist toward the finish line.

As for the sense of touch and feel on marathon day, there's the rub of petroleum jelly between toes, the stretch of soft cotton socks over ankles before sunrise, a moment of preparation to cherish. The feel of fabric on skin and the security of trainers wrapped around your feet (unless you're running barefoot, which, amazingly, some people do). There is the grip of a water bottle like a gun for protection, then the shoulder-to-shoulder huddle of the masses, along with hand-shaking, back-slapping and the general feel of being in the moment. Later will come the feel of cool water washing your face and pouring down the back of your neck.

There are also tastes to be savoured. Fresh soft bananas and sticky energy drinks on your lips; cool water on your throat; there are wine gums and jelly beans being offered in the closing miles, the sugar rush to help you toward the end.

As for the sights, I gaze at the clamour of colourful running vests, a river of causes rising up against suffering and illness and injustice, sweeping the streets with hope and purpose; people's heads of all generations and nations, dipping and rising, arms waving crazily, ponytails swinging, and today even the sun shining; home-made banners and hand-painted greetings of 'Run Mummy Run!' hanging from tree branches, and toddlers perched on fences; smiles, yes, so many smiles, and tears too, as thousands of aching bodies fold and bend and fall, hobbling hopefully towards the finish line. Each runner is the star of their own movie in the making.

The marathon, for thousands of people the world over, is a festival of life. From London to Loch Ness, from Tokyo to Tromso, it carries a kind of magic, uniting diverse communities who with their feet declare that they're not done just yet. Here, we become One. There is so much defiance at the start. There will be so much relief at the finish. But what of the miles in between? What of the story that joins the two?

It takes me 9 minutes to cross the start line behind the thousands of runners who were in the pens before me. Bill and the young lad inch forward alongside, nerves building, sun beaming.

No sooner have I crossed the start line, after a sharp turn through the stone pillars, than I see a line of thirty men, by the roadside, their backs to us. They're all having a pee. It seems they can't wait for the finish line for some relief. I join them and return to the race a few grams lighter. Will it be the crucial difference between a 4-hour finish time or not? Time will tell.

The miles click by, passing under yellow and green arches of balloons at each mile, in keeping with the sponsor Flora's colour scheme. I high-five kids at the roadside along Charlton Park Road and scoop up jelly beans from ice-cream tubs held out by pensioners in deckchairs. I'm wondering how much water will be enough to stave off dehydration, but also aware that too much water is even more harmful. 'Drink according to thirst,' my uncle has said, so this is what I do. I turn after the 3-mile marker into Woolwich Church Street.

Whack! Thwack, crack, crash...!

'Hmmmph!'

'Oi – stop it, you morons!' Bill yells. His ankle seems to be holding up, but we are under attack.

Ahead of us runners are slinging water bottles as high in the air as they can, somersaulting them over their shoulders so that they inevitably obey the laws of gravity and land on top of the runners – us – behind them. Bottles keep raining from the sky. I lose Bill in the melee, and to this day I don't know if he finished, as I never noted his race number.

I pass the *Cutty Sark* after 6 miles, boarded up for restoration and about to be decimated by a fire within a month of this marathon. The route wiggles towards Rotherhithe at mile 10 and the heat starts to claim runners. The collective pace slows. Heads go down. I run across Tower Bridge after mile 12, and am captivated by a huge airship hovering above. I wonder what their perspective of this marathon is. What if I could whizz all the way up there and just Take It All In? How does THIS look from up THERE? Runners like marching ants? Like white cells in the bloodstream? I reach halfway and look at my watch. Exactly 2 hours. It doesn't take long to do the sums and realise a 4-hour finish time is in the balance.

At mile 14 along The Highway I see the elite runners heading in the opposite direction, on the other side of the road. The noise is solid, more penetrating than oxygen. Team Macmillan Cancer Support cheer me on, waving green flags and inflatable batons. Another mile. Then another. As I climb East Ferry Road at mile 17 my body feels like the handbrake is on. The miles seem to be spreading themselves further and further apart when I'm not looking.

At mile 19 I hear my name from familiar voices and veer across the road. I hug my wife, my legs like raspberry jelly, red and unstable, and I forget the speech I'd prepared. The heat is in my skull as I carry on, disrupting my thoughts. My feet drag until I crumple to the road, like a tower of wooden Jenga blocks when too many pieces have been taken away. The pleasure-adrenalin of seeing my family has dissipated, now it's just me, swallowed by noise, waiting to be spewed out. As runners pass they pat my hunched back as I melt into The Embankment. The sun invades everything. Some speak condolences, others tread on my hands, not caring that I have become human roadkill. Someone stops and asks me how I am, forfeiting their personal-best time, but I... have... no... words. I am bent over, ready to be sick, less than 2 miles from the finish line. Everyone has their tipping point, an invisible marker beyond which the unknown is like a dark abyss, and from which you fear you may never return.

Then something happens which causes the mental fog to lift. 'CHRIS!' A stranger by Waterloo Bridge shouts at me. 'CHRIS!'

He can obviously read the wobbly white letters ironed onto my T-shirt. The bridge is swarming with supporters. They are on top, underneath, climbing inside it, like wasps to a fizzy drink. A nest of noise, energy fizzing. I look up, through my tears. I had been reading the biro on my forearm, where in capital letters I'd written 'FOR MUM. FOR DAVID'. The ink smudged but still readable.

'CHHRRRIIISSSSS!!' he yells. Runners thunder past my sunken body. He screams at me, for me, as if screaming his energy into me.

'CHRIS!! You can do this! You can do THIS!' His words are repetitive, incisive, and I notice the beautiful intonation, the word THIS like the bang of a gun. If ever you find yourself at the roadside of a marathon, behind the fence, cheer your heart out for those struggling in the final miles. It can be the difference between a broken dream and what they do next.

I grit my teeth and pull myself up from the sticky road. I try to see my temporary number-one fan, but he's just a voice absorbed in the crowd. I raise my chin, take two stumbling steps forward and then sprint. At mile 24 of the marathon I sprint for as long as I can, desperate for the damn thing to be over and done with. I run like I'm being electrocuted, yelling as I go, runners turning their heads as they see me surging through the pack. Half a mile later I collapse again, proving I have no sense. The final mile and a half takes me nearly 20 minutes.

Sir Arthur Conan Doyle was at the finish line of the London Olympics marathon in 1908, the first time the peculiar distance of 26.2 miles was run as a race, fixed for the convenience of the British Royal Family so they could watch the start and finish from the comfort of their own home.

'It is horrible, yet fascinating,' he wrote after witnessing the epic struggle of Italian baker Dorando Pietri to reach the finish line, 'this struggle between a set purpose and an utterly exhausted frame.' (Pietri was the first to finish that day, but he was disqualified because well-wishers had helped him up as he repeatedly fell over on the final stretch.)

My struggle between purpose and exhaustion includes weeping the last drops of grief onto a busy London road, my mind racing with memories. Exhaustion eventually yielded to Purpose. Without the anonymous encouragement, my knees would have stayed glued to the road. I could have become a permanent art installation. Instead I stumble to the finish, completing my first marathon in 4 hours 8 minutes.

After crossing the finish line I walk towards the railings, overcome with fatigue.

'Excuse... me... I... think I'm... going...' is as much as I say before I'm scooped into a wheelchair. Minutes later I'm lying on a mat in a St John Ambulance tent with a saline drip and blurred vision.

'Chris, do you know where you are?' someone keeps asking, looming over my prostrate body. Like hundreds of runners that day, I don't look my finest and I spend a queasy hour in the medical tent. When I'm told I can go, I hobble out, clueless as to where my family are. I finally locate them and sob on my dad's shoulder, the veil of unspoken loss now torn away. I lean on my wife as we descend the steps to the London Underground and begin our journey home. Up and down all those wretched concrete stairs, train passengers smile at me with sympathy, seeing me with my tears and medal, grief now exchanged for tight calf muscles and the right to say, 'I've bloody well done it.'

I was aged 33 when I completed my first marathon. As novelist and keen runner Haruki Murakami said, this is the same age that Jesus Christ died and the same age that Scott Fitzgerald started to go downhill.

'That age may be a kind of crossroads in life,' he said. If that's the case, where would this crossroads lead?

A celebrity-city marathon like London can be one valid starting place to run. But going for a run that doesn't involve four safety pins and a number attached to your chest can be a starting place too. It's not just about where or how you run, or when, or who with, or even how far. But why.

A record number of runners finish London that day (35,674 to be precise). My uncle is one of them, finishing 21 minutes after me. He meets his family at Horse Guards Parade, the designated repatriation area. I intend to meet him for the chance to swap our race stories and say thank you for his encouragement and advice during the months of training. But I never find him. We somehow miss each other.

His family say that on more than one occasion he'd retire to a pub after the race, with a pint next to his elbow, neglected like a just-dumped girlfriend at a disco, and would sit head in hands, mourning the PB time he didn't get. Yet again. His weary mind straying from what he'd just accomplished, falling under a spell, and tumbling weak-kneed into a fantasy world of that next elusive perfect run. Running, full of big dreams and unfinished pints. But he wasn't too bothered about his finishing time in London this time, as he'd run the Paris Marathon the week before. Two marathons in a week at age 58.

'My plan in Paris was to do a sub-four-hour race but, as so often in my running career, I came undone in the final three miles. The heat got to me and I finished in four hours three minutes,' he said. In fact on six occasions he finished 5 minutes outside the 4-hour mark.

What is it author Phil Hewitt says about a runner's 'healthy dose of discontent'? It's 'the natural state for a runner who hasn't run his final race'.

COME TO YOUR SENSES

Take care of your body. It's the only place you have to live.

Jim Rohn

As a runner it's easy to take a strong healthy body for granted. Like a stocking full of wrapped presents on Christmas Day or electricity at the flick of a switch, these things are just THERE. The gifts of power, stride, gulp and grasp, ready to enjoy. It's much easier to notice how the body looks from day to day, rather than what it does. But when you become injured or unwell, that's when you appreciate afresh what it was doing for you out there, mile after mile. One thing my first marathon in 2007 introduced me to was how to look after my body in terms of diet, exercise and rest, and also how to notice it, how to pay closer attention to my senses within it. Now, 6 years later, teaming up with my uncle for the Brighton Marathon isn't just about the externals: accumulating miles to satisfy the boxes on the training plan; practising running at speed with a wheelchair; getting it upgraded and race-ready; doing the race; raising sponsorship; collecting a medal; having a photo. I can't say I understand why my uncle has this illness, not in the Great Scheme of Things. It seems a cruel irony for someone who pushed their body to the full in marathons to now be dealing with an illness which strips physical ability away, layer by layer. It's got my attention, the chance to consider the internals of life differently, to notice the ordinary wonderful things your body can do, whilst it can do them.

For many of the people I know living with MND, their diagnosis took a year or more. Much depends on how informed the doctor is – some may only come across a couple of incidences of MND in their career. Spotting the disease is not obvious. The clues of the disease are in the faltering mechanics of the body. It might be a soberly slurred sentence. An inability to grasp the salt shaker like usual. Hands not able to unfold a lottery ticket. Unable to tie shoelaces. Or, like my uncle, stumbling over repeatedly for no reason. These are ways people with MND have described their first symptoms. Things which appear innocuous, but for them have a devastating message about what abilities the body is going to lose first.

Lindy Jones describes in her memoir *The Voice in My Head Is Perfect* how the illness affected her and her family, her outlook on life and on her body too. In a quest to reconcile herself to what was happening to her body, she wrote herself a letter, which she kindly gave me permission to share:

Tuesday 13 March

Dear Body

Bad news, I'm afraid.

This time tomorrow you will be in hospital. This is because the muscles in your mouth and throat don't work properly anymore and if you don't have medical help you and I will starve to death.

You will have a plastic tube with a camera put down your throat, which will then snake through you and pop out of a small incision made in your stomach wall. Liquid food can then be fed straight into you so you won't have to worry about things getting stuck or worse, going into your windpipe.

I know, it sounds awful, doesn't it? I'm scared too, but I've been told that they give you lots of drugs to help.

This is what is known as a PEG, not a clothes peg, but a Percutaneous, Endoscopic, Gastronomy. Something that I never, ever, in our old life together imagined happening, because you have always been so reliable and healthy.

Please try not to be too upset, it means that we can live together for a little bit longer even though we can't eat Real Food. We should have celebrated our last meal together but, like so many last things, I didn't recognise the occasion at the time.

Body, I just wanted to tell you how sorry I am that I didn't appreciate you enough when you were healthy. I was always complaining about your fat stomach, depriving you of food in a lifetime's attempt to stay slim. How I wish that instead of eating cottage cheese on Ryvitas every lunchtime I had allowed you to have a big chunky peanut butter and banana sandwich washed down by sweet coffee and a piece of cake. What a selfish cow I was, leaving you hungry for so much of the time.

What I'm trying to tell you, Body, is that I should have loved you more. Should have realised what a truly amazing machine you are, marvelled at the way everything worked so perfectly together. Now each move, each step, you allow me to take is precious because, one day, Body, I know you are going to give up on me. The Motor Neurone Disease, which, like an uninvited guest, barged into our lives 18 months ago, is going to be the death of us, if you will pardon the expression.

I know, I am sad too. I miss your voice. I miss the person you allowed me to be, but we had some good times together, didn't we? Some great nights out, laughing with friends. I'm just really sorry that maybe I didn't care for you enough, cherish your beautiful curves and strong arms and legs. So dearest Body, this is my way of marking the last day of our PEG-free life, only, before I go, can I ask a favour? Please try and keep the muscles in your chest strong. I've noticed recently that you have started to become a little breathless and it's scaring me. Please, please give me another couple of years. Three would do, though five would be better but I know that's unlikely. I have already had two. Please fight your hardest, because one definitely is not enough.

Don't cry, I know this is hard for you, but we'll just have to learn to live with PEG. I mean, it's not as if we have any choice, do we?

Body, thank you for all the years of good health you have given me, and good luck for tomorrow.

Your friend and partner,
Lindy

'Body, thank you for...' How many ways are there of finishing that sentence? The body gets a pretty tough time of it. Body image is such big business after all, a frenzy of persuasion to pay more attention to what's not up to scratch (according to invented definitions), and what requires improvement, rather than to stand and stare and marvel at what we do have. When I stand in front of a hundred teenagers as part of my education work through my charity, and talk about the physical changes bodies go through during adolescence, they sit attentively, flushes of embarrassment on faces. They know I'm not talking about something abstract, but something they're residents in. Teenagers are acutely aware of how their bodies look, feel and smell.

Your body loves you. It keeps you alive when you sleep, clots your blood when you're cut, and gives you clues (called pain) about inside trouble. It is – you are – a work of art. Wonderfully made. No body is perfect or invincible. But every body is incredible, whatever its appearance.

If we realised what we are residents in, wouldn't it be the most natural thing in the world to want to discover what it's capable of, whilst the window of time is available to us?

I read Lindy's words and place her book down on the coffee table. I decide to experiment. Her letter has me thinking about the miraculous machinery of the body. What if I go for a run and just pay attention to that? *Not* the aches and pains like usual, but the rhythm, the motion, the sensations. To notice what's not the problem. It looks chilly outside, evening clouds approaching, a dark blanket across a turquoise sky. My marathon-training plan says a 9-mile tempo run, which inevitably includes hills. I've been doing more miles than expected of late, and will probably surpass the 120 miles planned for December. I fill my water bottle, pull on my long compression socks, then my running tights, and feel the hit of the elastic against my waist. I grab my hi-viz top and fluorescent gloves, then find my head-torch and armband with flashing red LEDs. I load up the Glympse application on my phone, which acts as a tracking device to selected recipients. There are no prizes for causing worry about your whereabouts, especially when running in the dark. I don't know why, but I laugh as I tie up the laces on my trainers. I'm analysing each action, but it's all too quick, too natural, and I forget there was a time when I had to learn all this. I step out the door and run through the village. My body launches into Automatic, bending, lifting, holding, reaching, stretching, contacting, compressing, absorbing, bounding, rising, propelling. Each step part of a chain reaction. I run faster, sensing the crescendo of action, the rhythm of my limbs moving piston-like, strength upon strength, tiny tender touches upon tarmac. I'm getting out of my head and into my body, and it's liberating.

I hear a shout as a car speeds past from behind me, half a head stuck out the passenger window. It sounds like 'You fascist-something or other'. My default mode is to want to hurl my water bottle at the rear windscreen, but I catch myself. I take a breath. I'm a sensitive soul, but I know the insults say more about them than me. I'd rather be in my body than theirs, so I pretend he said I'm the 'fastest-something or other' and, agreeing with the compliment, I find myself chuckling, relaxing back into the run and back into my body.

As I run, all I hear is breathing, all I see is stars.

For 8 of the 9 miles there isn't a single lamppost to light my way, just darkness, in all its intensity. This night thirsts for light. I feel overcome in seconds. I trust my head-torch to illuminate the next step, no further. Sometimes the next step is all you need.

I reach a disused railway line accessed through a creaking metal gate, and twist my body through, like a nifty dance move. I run past an old railway carriage, which serves as a cafe in summer but is a heap of rusting metal in winter. A train permanently stationed. I steam past. I admit I feel scared as my feet pierce the darkness, trainers scuffing stones and causing puffs of chalk to rise up like small explosions. My imagination escapes onto the black canvas and creates ridiculous scenarios. What's hiding in the bushes? Malevolent foxes with massive teeth preying on the loneliness of a long-distance runner? No, I don't feel lonely, but I'm entirely alone. Aloneness is different to loneliness. Solitude, not separation. It's so easy to get lost in thought, my mind detaching from my body. Suddenly they are following different routes, like an inversion of the London Marathon: one start line of thought fracturing into multiple finish lines. 'What if this? What if that?' There is a time to strategise, and there's a time to come back to where you are. Running doesn't have to mean rushing. We can create a different relationship with the run when we release ourselves from the relentless tick-tick-tick of time. Running helps me find mental stillness. My worry or stress is like a piece of a Tetris puzzle, jiggling and twisting inside me as I run, until it eventually finds its home, a place where it can settle for now. I can begin to see the issue for the intrusion or invitation it is. Perhaps a purpose emerges which is useful to me, but not always. A lot of the time it's just 'head stuff' to let go of, as if running a physical distance also creates a mental distance. Learning to not live in the past, pressing pause on Automatic, coming back to your senses. Switching from the go-getting, strategic-planning, list-conquering, door-locking, oven-turning-off part of the brain to just being present. Coming back to what you hear and see, smell, touch and taste. Senses are not thoughts. They don't have thought intrinsically attached to them; they are just the means by which you have contact with the world. Thoughts can be devilish travel agents – we have about 60,000 of them a day – taking you to places you never intended to go. But you can get a return ticket. When you pay attention to your senses – the smell of roses, splash of puddles, sight of starlings, sound of wind in trees – your thoughts get a rest. You get headspace. Your senses become a safety valve.

'Body, thank you for... putting me in touch with the environment in which I run and live.'

In tonight's December temperatures each breath is illuminated by my head-torch, creating a bright fog in front of me, like I'm leaking smoke. I can't see where I'm going, so I turn my head to the side to breathe, which is a nuisance because I need to look where I'm going.

I run to start again. I like starting again. The night is not permanent, it will not endure, there's always a new day ahead.

Every now and then I turn my head-torch off to be brave.

'Bravery is a choice you make, not a feeling you wait for,' my mum said, as ovarian cancer spread its pernicious fingers through her body. I look up and find the moon, a smudged light obscured by cloud. Is my mum watching tonight, from somewhere beyond?

I pick up the pace, feet fumbling over lonely stones, crunching discarded crisp packets. I listen to the soundtrack of the night. Rabbits leaping out of my way, bats slicing the fog above. There is a disco of creatures around me, out of view; the night is well and truly alive. I reach the place where I once saw a naked man clamber out of the bushes, but that was in summer when the train carriage cafe was still open, and the sun was slipping lazily out of the sky. I ran a fast mile in the opposite direction that evening, not knowing or trusting his intentions.

I try to let my feet and breathing fall into rhythm with each other, but it's clumsy. I want my mind to stay in one place, but my headspace is wayward. I try to focus on just the sounds I hear – the swish-whoosh of trees, the crrrr-crrrr of my feet on the gravel, but my mind has drifted. It's gone again. I reach the end of a track and clamber over a gate into a field. My numbing fingers wrap around the wet metal pole. Over I go, stepping onto each rung in turn, my feet flinging echoes into the night. I look into the apparent nothingness, a black veil, an invisible cloak. What will I find if I keep going? I'm running over earth which yields easily under my weight, this field has been churned by tractors. My footprints become a temporary signature of progress.

Sometimes our mental equilibrium tips the scales, our mood nosedives and our body then glues itself to the corner of the sofa.

'Body, thank you for...' well, what exactly? Only real people have heads knotted with loose ends. When I run, I remember it's OK to feel scared, stressed, furious. I run to feel the emotion, then remember it can pass, like the muddy footprints behind me.

I start laughing at the sound of wet mud clawing at my trainers, sucking at my heels as if trying to swallow me from beneath, pulling me into the throat of the earth. It sounds like an exaggerated kiss. My feet kissing the earth. Here I am, my body longing for movement, my mind desiring stillness, my feet seeking a connection to the ground. I run in search of this juxtaposition. In the dark it seems easier to find. After 8 miles my breathing sounds like I'm a hunted man, but I'm the one who is searching, pursuing the present moment.

I reach the edge of the field on my way home and pause before twisting through the metal gate. I look up. I can see things in the dark I couldn't in the light. The immensity of the night sky, cluttered with constellations like shining graffiti, so close, like it's leaning towards me, as if to whisper some vital truth. To remind me I am here, in my body, and not to be so lost in thought. To be present. The sky reminds me something greater is going on than my own small story. It doesn't make sense isolated on its own. Perhaps our stories are like stars, brighter when we look to their edges, when we notice the far grander constellations to which they – and we – belong. Stories connected, not by made-up lines on an astrologer's map, but in the context of the darkness in which they shine.

I have a mile to get home... I start running faster. 'Body, thank you...'

All I.
Hear is.
Breathing.
All I.
See is.
Stars.

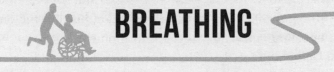

BREATHING

Every parting gives a foretaste of death; every reunion a hint of the resurrection.

Arthur Schopenhauer

Seventy-three minutes. That's how long it was. Seventy-three minutes of putting the gift of a life under the microscope.

Reading Lindy's and the Reverend Michael Wenham's memoirs of life with MND, to help me understand what's yet to come for my uncle, has me sensitised to anything to do with the illness, like when you want a new car and suddenly the only car that seems to be on the road is the model you're after.

I first knew about the film whilst walking through a whitewashed London Underground tunnel towards the Bakerloo Line. Massive curved posters with a man, Neil Platt, pictured in a wheelchair on them. The film title in bold across the top: *I Am Breathing*. In front of the poster, a saxophone player was busking, the sound of the blues curling and filling the tunnel like smoke vapours. There was the chink-chink of coins being thrown in to his instrument case by commuters in a hurry. On Automatic.

Tonight I saw the film in my lounge, a life playing out on the screen. Next to it stood our Christmas tree, bereft of decorations or gifts beneath its branches.

Neil, a lover of motorbikes and dad to a 2-year-old boy, Oscar, was 33 when he was diagnosed with MND. He wanted to capture as much of life as he could for his son, wondering what questions his son would ask him if he were to live long enough to find out.

'Of what importance have my thirty-three years of life been?' he asked.

Neil was diagnosed in 2007 after falling over inexplicably more and more often, and died 2 years later. Thirty-three years, 'a kind of crossroads,' said Murakami. Neil's dad had died of the same disease when Neil was 22. Only in a minority of cases, about one in twenty, is MND hereditary. The award-winning film is testament to Neil's bravery and insight, and to that of his wife Louise and family.

I thought of my uncle as I watched the seasons on screen change, and Neil's physical strength deteriorate. Perhaps that physical strength was internalised and transferred into greater mental resolve? As my uncle's illness advances, his breathing is becoming more laboured and his right arm hangs limply at his side so he can no longer drive. Or hug fully. Holding cutlery is trickier now. It won't improve.

The final scene showed Neil with his wife, dictating his hundredth and final blog entry. Each word spoken between ventilator-assisted breaths. Tears striping their cheeks. These were their last moments together at home before going to the hospice for, as Neil put it, 'kicking-out time'.

The film was sobering and sad, yet also a triumph of the ordinary moments of a life. As Neil wrote in his blog, 'You could do me a favour – don't let yours slip by unnoticed.' I'm sorry, Neil, but sometimes we do. Sometimes the morning has gone before we have greeted it. Sometimes golden leaves are trodden underfoot and we ignore what they herald, another year assigned to the treasure chest, another year waiting to be worn like a crown.

I watched and wept at the simplicity of Oscar stroking his daddy's immobile hand, looking at his dad, then out the window at the motionless swing, perhaps wondering why his dad didn't whisk him up and take him outside. Father and son, side by side. I thought of my own dad. I thought of Mick and Phil. Uncle Andrew and Paul. Then I think about my own sons, both sleeping. Our time as fathers is so precious. How much do I let slip by unnoticed? What would happen if I paused now and then, and marvelled at the blinks, the beats, the breaths that fill our moments together? Must I hurry through my life? Why do I let those things which seem so urgent squash what is truly important?

Earlier in the day my son Caleb and I had worked on our allotment. I brought along the spade, shovel and rake. He brought a plastic bag full of Haribo sweets and Drumstick lollipops. I had dropped a couple of shining apples in the bag to keep Mummy happy.

Knowing the temperature was set to drop, I wanted to get as much of the allotment dug over as I could before terra firma became terra even firmer. As we approached the dirty maze of allotment patches, a man dashed across the empty car park towards me by the village hall, adjacent to the allotments.

'We have a coffee morning on, you know, with tea and cake, oh, and a tombola,' he said.

The car park was generously decorated with orange balloons, the words 'Myeloma UK' printed on each of them. He'd gone to a lot of trouble but the car park indicated people had other things to do. The coffee morning that served tea was slipping by unnoticed. I watched him pace back and forth, like an expectant dad in a hospital corridor.

I spent the morning digging and thinking about him. Wondering if the line separating us had been erased by the shared experience of loss. I glanced over at the empty car park. As I turned the soil, exposing new layers, something in me was disturbed. What was his connection with the orange-ballooned charity? A survivor himself of bone marrow cancer perhaps? Or someone in his family? I wondered what our conversation would be if we sat down over a cup of tea and breathed our stories of loss, resuscitating them with memory. Creating different endings perhaps. Which parts would we pull out and discard? Suffering connects us with others in ways nothing else can. It gets our attention, shifts us out of Automatic.

My son balanced on the spade as if it were a pogo stick, wobbling it to and fro in the claggy soil. I picked out weeds like Brussels sprouts from a Christmas dinner.

'Daddy, can we have something to eat?' he said.

We'd been working for 10 minutes. I checked my pockets with thoughts of getting a cup of tea and chancing it on the tombola, but I was out of change. Instead we sat down under the canopy of the walnut tree and unwrapped two Drumstick lollies.

'OK, let's cut back the raspberry canes next,' I said. My son leapt up.

'Oh cool, I know how to use the scissors, Daddy.'

'Secateurs,' I corrected him, knowing it wouldn't make the slightest difference, but that's what we parents do. We tweak and advise to keep our kids on the straight and narrow of correct vocabulary. A waste of breath, it so often feels. 'I'll cut. You stack,' I said.

I grasped the prickled stems of the raspberry canes, and cut them near the earth, missing the new shoots. Who knows if there will be fruit on them next summer, nearly 8 months away. A whole life cycle from conception to first shoots. We are late in the year for doing this. Why do I feel like I'm so often trying to catch up with my life? I passed bundles of cut canes to Caleb, he grabbed them and raced to the compost heap, then back again, competing with me, a grin on his face.

'LOOK, DADDY!!' he shouted. He'd discovered a paving slab buried amongst the canes. We levered it up with a spade, both of us breathing noisily with the dead weight of it, then rolled it across the allotment, like cavemen trying out the world's first wheel.

That moment there. Father and son, side by side, cartwheeling a paving slab, clothed in age with a missing corner, across clumpy earth. We stopped and looked at each other halfway, as if acknowledging the moment. Then it was gone. Moments don't stick around, but memories do.

How many ordinary things were happening on the allotment that Neil Platt would have loved to have done with his son in a few years, but couldn't? If he'd been there his skin would have felt the cold air; his fingers could have sensed the weight of the stone; his feet would have known the solid earth beneath him; he would have smelled the wet earth. Although his senses remained intact, his motor neurones undid his capability to dig, grip, stand, unwrap a lollipop and chew it. It's easy to forget to feel the earth at our fingertips and smell all that wonder which passes under our noses. Simple sensory pleasures, lost. For Neil swallowing and speaking gradually became impossible. Then it was 'time at the bar, ladies and gentlemen', as he put it.

Seeing Neil in the film tonight was a chance to look at my life differently, through the lens of limited time. A reminder that life is not a waste of breath. Presence matters for its own sake. In a sense the film wasn't about mourning what is lost, but unwrapping what is before your eyes.

With the allotment jobs done, I went for a weekend run of 10 miles, not mindful of the biomechanics of each step and of what my body was doing without my conscious intervention. I went running on Automatic. I got lost along country lanes in the dusk and ended up sprinting 11 miles to get back home in time for the village Christmas lights switch-on. I burst through the door in my fluorescent yellow kit, sounding like I'd been chased by the police. I gasped for breath, lurched into the kitchen and ate cake without tasting it. I pounded upstairs for a shower two steps at a time, not appreciating my power. I didn't notice the water on my skin. I was ready to go out again with seconds to spare, standing by the door, triumphantly exhausted. Totally missing the moment, but at least I could tick another long run off my training plan.

'Dear Body, thank you for putting up with me even when I ignore you.'

Perhaps this is why I write. To chronicle something of these days of ordinary wonder, moments of eating sticky lollipops under a walnut tree, listening to the territorial song of the robin, side by side with my son. Of Presence before Absence. To not let it all slip by... unnoticed, accepting I won't ever figure out of what importance it all is. As author Mitch Albom says, perhaps this is why we want there to be a life after this one, to make better sense of our time on earth.

As I emerged that day from the Bakerloo Line, having seen the poster and breathed in the melancholy of the jazz, I ran up the stairs into London Paddington train station. I stood under the departures board as it struggled to make up its mind about which platform my train would leave from. WAITING… WAITING. I looked around, taking in the scene. It was Friday evening; over two hundred people were tucked in behind me. Men with long beards, pensioners in trilby hats, women nursing babies, teenagers on smartphones, couples yawning away their long day and muttering weekend plans, sipping from polystyrene cups. I tried counting the nationalities represented: Malaysian, French, American, Sri Lankan, Welsh. Just guessing at how much of the earth was waiting to depart.

'What do we all have in common here?' I wondered. 'We all look so different. But what joins us?' The status for the 19:22 still flickered; as I waited, it became obvious. We were all breathing the same air, connected by the same dependency. The oxygen was in all of us and all of us were in the oxygen. None of us owned that air. No one could brand it, copyright it, tax it, trade it. There is no Them and Us.

Pause now. Notice your breath. For a few seconds just listen to your breathing, arriving and leaving. Notice the blink of your eyes. And then… the beat of your heart. Notice the ground beneath your feet rising up to hold you. As you do, you will notice the power of stillness pulsing inside you. This is happening every second of every day you're here. You are in your life, and life is in you.

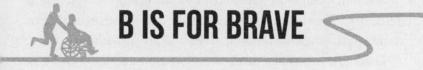

B IS FOR BRAVE

How lucky I am to have something that
makes saying goodbye so hard.

A. A. Milne

Esther laughs. Loudly. Even whilst telling the story of dealing with her dad in his final months of living with motor neurone disease.

I had met Esther about a year before, when we were trying to move house. She'd been looking at a house for her mum, which we had put an offer on. As things turned out neither of us bought that particular house, but we kept crossing paths in Stratford-upon-Avon in various shops and would ask how each other was getting on with the house move. Soon other connections came to light, including a mention of her dad's illness. I admitted I didn't know very much about it but wanted to find out more.

'Well, if you want to know more why don't we get a coffee?' she said. 'It's important you know what it's really like.'

The invitation came at the start of my learning curve about the illness, and halfway into my wheelchair-marathon training in late 2012. Learning and running, hand in hand.

We meet in a tea shop that sells everything but coffee. I arrange all the cups and pots in front of us like a game of chess, feeling nervous about the conversation to come.

'My dad thought he had sciatica for about four years,' Esther tells me. 'Three years before he died he had neurological symptoms, you know, falling over and stuff, without reason.'

There are points like this I can relate to immediately because of how the illness is affecting my uncle. Other things are an eye-opener. This is striking out into unfamiliar territory, but I want to understand the reality of the disease.

'Oh my, it took so long to get a diagnosis,' she says. 'I was on my knees pleading with the consultant to make the diagnosis. Being a biochemist myself, being able to read the clinical jargon, I knew the score, but to actually get them to commit to a diagnosis took too long.'

'How did you respond to knowing your dad had MND?' I ask.

'Oh, it was such a relief after what we'd been through. My dad asked the consultant how long before the illness killed him. The consultant said "Er... three years." When my dad pressed him, the consultant relented, "Probably less, probably a lot less." And it was. Five months, to be precise.'

Allan wasn't actually Esther's birth father. Her dad died when she was four, and Allan came into her life when she was six.

'I fell in love with Allan straight away. Stepdad doesn't really describe it. To me he was my dad,' she says.

Esther slurps her soup, as the tea shop fills up, then continues.

'It was a relief when he finally got a wheelchair. Before he accepted his condition, it was tough emotionally for him, and tough physically for everyone else. Even with the wheelchair it could take my mother and me an hour to transfer him from his armchair to his wheelchair then to the stairlift, then back to his wheelchair to take him to his bed upstairs. Imagine that. It was hard for him, and hard for us too. Yeah, it was frustrating. To be fair, it made us angry and in those quiet moments by ourselves it made us cry.' I sit and nod as Esther wipes her eyes liberally with the cafe napkin.

'You just get on with it,' she says, shrugging and throwing her hands up, thankfully not with a cup of tea in her hand. 'Knowing our time to do normal things was drawing to an end, I took him for lunch at the pub. After we'd eaten, I pushed him in his wheelchair out into the car park, and there was a man up a ladder painting the outside of the pub. He stopped and watched us.'

Esther starts chuckling. 'He was watching me wrestling with my dad, trying to get him from the wheelchair into the car. It looked,' she pauses for a moment, 'very inappropriate. Me straddling my dad. The painter called out, "Do you want a hand, love?" For some reason I said, "I think I've mastered the position, thanks!" What was I thinking?' Esther is laughing so loudly everyone in the tea shop can hear her story. I'm not sure whether to be embarrassed or to appreciate how we often use humour to protect ourselves.

Esther continues. 'Motor neurone disease is tough because you have to face the inevitable. It's a roller-coaster ride even though you know the end result. You often find yourself explaining your loved one has MND because of their lack of mobility or awkward speech. Shop assistants giving you funny looks and that kind of thing. Usually people say "Oh that's a terrible condition." One day you feel like shouting back, "Yes, thank you for the reminder, there's nothing we can do to take this thing away." Other days, you smile and say, "You're right, but we're doing the best we can, thank you." Strangely, good things can come from it,' she says.

She puts down her cup. There is a pause as she adjusts herself on the seat.

'You know, Chris, I can tell you that my relationship with my dad went incredibly deep in those closing months. You have to tackle life and death's tough decisions together. You have to be brave, and in being brave together, you connect in a way life wouldn't usually allow. Through the heartache, frustration and anger, with some courage, you can find something precious.'

I think stories like Esther's are there to reach us, and then teach us something. With MND, the inevitability of death does lurk closer, it arrives sooner, perhaps it approaches more menacingly because of the way it wastes the muscles even as the mind stays razor sharp. But there is the chance to be brave and let life still flourish, just differently.

In his memoir of facing the illness, the Reverend Michael Wenham says he learned to value life 'frame by frame', discovering a new fascination with intricately woven spiders' webs, and strutting chickens. Life didn't become one continual decline into misery, even though he had a life-limiting diagnosis. He says although there are times when despair washes over you, it doesn't have to become the focal point. Life can still be noticed and enjoyed, just more slowly.

Talking about the end of life doesn't bring it closer. It's not easy to face, for anyone, we all have an instinct to survive.

Perhaps that's why we prefer to read about death or watch it in films, keep it at arm's length, rather than talk about it. Talking makes it feel real. Perhaps that's why we give death other names: passed away; moved on; crossed the great divide; left these shores. Talking as if death were a sailing trip.

'So how were those closing days?' I ask, leaning back on the padded chair, adjusting to the spices in my drink.

She looks up.

'There was a changing point when we had to start assuming my dad couldn't do something rather than assume he could. He was a brave man by nature; he was of that generation that got on with things. He told us, "When I can't feed myself, that's when the condition has got the better of me." Yes, he was a brave man.'

I hear echoes of my mum in those words, 'being brave is a choice, not a feeling.' I don't know if 'brave' is a default setting we are born with. I think along our lifeline we get chances to notice it, learn how it feels a little, to choose it more often. Chances like our first toddling steps, our first taste of green vegetables, the first time we jump off the third stair or risk a kiss at the school disco. Perhaps all these are tiny practice steps towards a time in our lives when being brave has to start with a capital 'B'. When it's not just broccoli we face, but something more serious.

'What about, you know, practical stuff for your dad?' I ask. I scribble notes like a trainee journalist. My black book is getting plump.

'We got things like a gel seat for his wheelchair because he was sat in it for a long time. In the later stages when the illness affected his breathing, one practical thing was a torso support to make breathing easier.'

I do my best to imagine a torso support on an adult male, but I don't find it easy. MND affects people very differently, so getting an independent assessment from an occupational therapist is the best course of action. It avoids making expensive mistakes, as there is equipment that can improve comfort and portability, but individuals need to know what is best for them.

Some people with the illness show unexpected behavioural changes. The MND Association list these as 'restlessness, acting impulsively, eating lots of sweet foods, lacking drive, fixating on one activity or routine, or lacking empathy for others'. There can be a variety of causes for these, perhaps breathing problems causing fatigue, frustration as disability increases, chest or urinary infections leading to confusion. For some there is a symptom called emotional lability, where laughing or crying happens at inappropriate times. This can be disorienting.

Many have benefitted from new technology. It can't reverse the disease, but it can help people to stay connected to who and what they love more meaningfully. Sarah Ezekiel is an artist who no longer has the powers of grasp or speech. She was aged 34 when diagnosed with MND, with a newborn baby and a 3-year-old child. Within a year she couldn't use her hands. Now, through the use of a Tobii Eye Tracker, she creates, painting with her eyes.

'Eyegaze technology has given me a new lease of life,' she told me by email. Written with her eyes. 'I feel more complete being able to create again. I always wanted to be an artist and Eyegaze has enabled me to fulfil that dream.'

The technology means she can also open her front door, use Facebook and contact her carers. Sarah controls a computer cursor with just her eye, looking at a specific point on the screen, communicating by spelling out words and sentences on a virtual keyboard. 'I want people to understand that there's always hope and everything is possible.'

'Everything is possible.' That's a staggering mindset to hold in the face of a terminal illness which late historian Tony Judt described as like being 'confined to an iron suit, cold and unforgiving… a prison which is shrinking by six inches each day'. My uncle's illness has introduced me to a community of people on social media like Sarah who have radically challenged my view of the body, mind and time. Until this unexpected journey, I had never fathomed the bravery and triumph of the human spirit.

Esther continues. 'My dad had three months with a nippy.'

I obviously look puzzled, because she flaps her hand at me in a kind-of 'okaaaaay, let me explain' manner. It's a miracle nothing on our table has been knocked over.

'Someone with MND can't have an oxygen mask because of carbon monoxide poisoning, so the nippy forces the diaphragm to move without adding oxygen,' she explains.

Later at home I do a search on the Internet for 'MND nippy'. I learn that experiencing breathing difficulties is a cruel part of the closing stages of MND, because the disease reduces the muscle strength to do this automated action normally. Choking fits can be both tiring and frightening. One piece of simple equipment can help. A 'nippy' (or NPPV) in full is a 'non-invasive positive pressure ventilation'. This small machine supports the person's own breathing by providing extra air through a face mask or nasal tubes. For some it helps them sleep better and speak easier, but it can take time to get used to, including for those caring for people with MND.

Equipment such as this is what some of our fundraising will be going towards.

'We wrote a plan with my dad. I guess a bit like people have a birth plan,' Esther says. 'It made decisions easier when it came to it.'

Plans? PLANS!? I think to myself. We plan for births, weddings, holidays and career moves. We plan marathon training and what outfit to wear to the restaurant, a week in advance if you're like my wife. When does anyone plan positive decisions to do with the very end of their life? Of course, people are actually doing this all the time. My brother-in-law Graham is a funeral director and helps people prepare for the end; I've just been turning a blind eye.

'Dying is just as important as being born,' say the MND Association. 'The person's ability to communicate often shrinks as the illness progresses, sometimes rapidly, so it's good to think through practical things in advance. Not all in one go, though.' Esther is a reminder that we never stop being humans who sometimes feel scared, cross and tired. One action at a time was her strategy.

Plans can provide reassurance and a sense of choice, some control when so many other things are happening beyond your control. Frustration and sadness are normal, for the person with MND as well as family and friends. But people's emotions aren't synchronised, so permission to express emotion is important, whether speaking it or writing it down. Our emotions aren't the totality of who we are. There's a difference between 'I am depressed' and 'I feel depressed', one suggesting permanence, the other transience. We have emotions about what matters to us, they indicate our values, a sign of what and whom we love. No emotion is negative. Unpleasant emotion? Sure. Awkward, puzzling and inconvenient? Yep. But all emotions have some usefulness; they all provide some kind of insight into what's going on within us. Making plans, choosing to do the best you can with what you have and know, are brave steps towards acceptance.

The queue in the tea shop is lengthening and the noise level is rising. People are mulling over the menu; black tea, green tea, white tea, blue tea. I never knew there was blue tea. People planning their choice as they unzip coats, remove scarves and collapse umbrellas.

I've filled several pages of my notebook, but there's always a question which I come back to.

'How did you cope?' I ask.

'You don't think about coping, you just keep going. MND is unpredictable. Things change not when you expect them to.' Esther is very direct. She tells me some things didn't go to plan, but it was still good to have the plan. No person's story is a linear journey from A to B. Introduction, Middle, Conclusion, like a school essay.

Perhaps making plans in the face of a life-limiting illness is one way that the fear and mysteries around death are faced. Later at home I record some of the things in my book, inspired by Esther:

Do practical things, including making a will.

Get equipment that, if possible, makes things more comfortable.

Enjoy time together. Go out for lunch when you can, but not where there's a painter halfway up a ladder.

THE REASON I RUN

Write your wishes down so you know they're known, especially if the ability to communicate is reducing as normally happens with MND.

Sort out your money affairs (for peace of mind).

Talk about tricky things little bits at a time. Not in one go.

I add one more of my own:

Believe there's a bigger story than your own.

But that's not all. There's one extra, one that takes bravery, plus a pen and paper.

'The family all wrote goodbye letters to Dad,' Esther says. 'Saying whatever they wanted to say. They weren't really long letters, just honest. It was our way of saying goodbye while my dad could understand. He read them all a week before he died.' Esther sits upright with her cup resting on her lap. There is silence between us. It gives me a chance to consider it. The power of a letter to say thank you, and I forgive you, and I love you. A 'good' goodbye letter.

Then the *BBC News* theme tune bursts to life on the television behind us. The familiar rhythmic beeping, a clock ticking down. Ironic really, because I have a headline right here about a family that faced the cruelty of MND, and reached in and rescued from its grasp a great armful of love.

As Saint Augustine said, 'Hope has two beautiful daughters: anger and courage. Anger at the way things are, and courage to see that they do not remain as they are.'

Esther shakes her head.

'Tell you what, though, we were right naffed off Dad never said anything back to us!' and she laughs again, slapping the table with her hand, my empty cup jolting with surprise. People look over at us.

It's not comfortable having conversations like this, but they are necessary and strengthen my motivation. I feel privileged to have heard Esther's story. There was no self-indulgence, just the honesty and clarity that comes through dark times. Her laughter is a reminder that a story continues beyond the sadness.

I'm late getting home, my marathon-training schedule for this past week is at risk of going on strike, but I'll squeeze a quick run in before picking the kids up from school if I can. A chance to process the stories I'm hearing, as long as nothing goes wrong on the way.

GENERATION GAME

*If everything seems under control then
you're not going fast enough.*

Mario Andretti

I walk through my front door and dash straight upstairs to grab my not-quite-dry running kit from the radiator and put it on. I don go-faster striped mittens on our youngest son, Toby, and buckle him into his three-wheeled buggy. Everything has to be done quickly. In winter drizzle, and with just half an hour to spare before picking my other two kids up from school, we set off for a quick 4-mile run-and-push around the village. The first mile is a ridiculous sub-8-minute pace as my adrenalin levels are going crazy, the last is even faster and more perilous, because I realise I'm going to be late to the school gates for pick-up time. There's nothing like a deadline and public criticism from your children to spur you on. Given my uncle lives nearly 150 miles away, I figure I have to grab every chance I can to run pushing anyone and anything.

This run is a bonus, crowbarred in as an extra to my training plan. The plan dictates just four runs a week as my wife is training for the London Marathon and we have to juggle childcare, with a week of reduced mileage each month to help prevent injury. My 'drop week' is usually half the mileage. The plan also outlines a strict daily routine of single leg squats, lunges, 30 sit-ups, 30 press-ups, and planks for as long as I can hold them. But I don't like core-strength work, so I might delegate all this out to my wife as an early Christmas present. The twist for this plan which makes it different to all my previous ones is the need to seize pushing, well, anything I find. Our youngest son cannot refuse as he doesn't yet have words like 'No way!' and 'You must be kidding!' at his disposal. But he also comes with a mode of transport included. In hindsight, I wish I'd insured his pushchair.

I encounter a few problems whilst out running-pushing that are not obvious when running solo.

Firstly, pavement parking by vans (usually), where there has been zero consideration for pushchairs and wheelchairs. I have to slow down and twist the pushchair at strange angles every 20 metres as I run up a residential street in order not to leave scratch marks down the side of the vans. Tempted though I am.

Secondly, running and pushing a pushchair single-handedly whilst rehydrating is not something they teach you at school. Picture head tilted back, swigging freely from a water bottle, pushchair careering wildly from left to right. This is a tricky matter, causing large wet patches all down my front and looks of concern regarding incontinence from passers-by.

Today, in my exuberance, as I cross a road the pushchair hits the kerb. I realise I'm lying on top of the pushchair, which has somersaulted itself over onto the pavement. Somewhere under there is Toby. I've cut my ankles and elbows but the pushchair is intact. So is my son. He didn't want to get out, maybe frozen with fear. He and Dennis should swap notes.

Although runners are used to looking like a fashion crash, turning heads for all the wrong reasons, arriving at the school gates the way I did should be outlawed. I'm sweating, breathing heavily and wearing mud-splattered, skin-tight leggings with fluorescent streaks across the hip. I have blood on my elbows. 'Hello kids!'

***

Whereas Toby is one and a half years old and can't yet articulate his wishes to escape when I am at the handlebars of his buggy, my other new training partner is 91 and a half years old and should know better. From one end of the generation spectrum to the other.

Whilst enjoying a weekend away with all my wife's family to celebrate my mother-in-law's sixtieth birthday, we venture a grand day out together at Warwick Castle. It's December, but the sky is July-blue. Has someone turned the year on its head? It's a very public opportunity to train, with all my wife's family there, and family friends. My father-in-law lifts the wheelchair out from the boot of his car.

'So who wants to push then?' he says. My father-in-law has a very loud voice, even when he's whispering. At that point anyone in Warwickshire had the chance of volunteering to push Great Grandma.

'Yep, I will,' I say, sounding a little too enthusiastic, a glint in my eye about what was to come.

I think it's safe to say Great Grandma will remember this particular day in her wheelchair forever. She will recollect being zoomed for multiple laps around the castle courtyard, at full tilt, the front wheels of her wheelchair rattling and vibrating as if penetrating the speed barrier. I recall Mick's hands doing that impression of wiggly fishes to warn me of their probable delinquency. Castle visitors leap out the way. They point fingers and cameras at us as her spotted woolly blanket flaps in the wind. Tourists check their glossy Warwick Castle brochures for which attraction we might be. One lady applauds as we speed by, a nonagenarian and her handler out for a spin.

After thanking me for pushing her around the grounds, past the falconry display and the stocks with 'Village Idiot' painted on them, she confesses she thought she 'looked a bit like a twit'. Sorry, Great Grandma. Your revenge is I had tight calf muscles the following day, and a speeding ticket from the Dungeon Master. It's also clear that pushing an NHS wheelchair at speed with the small handles facing back at you is very uncomfortable. Even shopping trolleys are more comfortably designed. I note that something must be done about this.

As a result of our training run together, Great Grandma becomes the first person to sponsor us and I'm touched by her generosity. Something changes in my connection with her. I want to know more of her story, now she's put her heart rate on the line for me. It seems speeding around Warwick Castle courtyard in a wheelchair is a new way of breaking down generational barriers. What other connections are there beneath the surface?

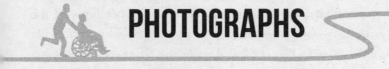# PHOTOGRAPHS

No story lives unless someone wants to listen.

J. K. Rowling

January arrives and doesn't seem happy about it, lines of drizzle score the windscreen as my family and I drive to Great Grandma's house. The clouds have slumped themselves down for the day. In Roman mythology, Janus (after which January is named) was the god of beginnings and transitions and was often depicted as having two faces, one looking back, the other forward. Pretty handy for reverse-parking, or doing the Macarena. I think back over the last 6 months. I feel I've come so far – learning about MND through personal stories, training with wheelchairs, banking hundreds of miles of running, and meeting inspirational people along the way. Now it's 2013, the year of our marathon. There still seems such a long way to go. Do we look back more as we get older? How do we make sense of life?

Visiting Great Grandma at her Bedfordshire bungalow, I take in the photographs populated on every shelf and mantelpiece, curious about all the stories. There are four generations of family on show. It's like a story told backwards, pictures of toothy children in high-definition colour at the front, photographs of adults with bad haircuts sheltering in rows behind, through to faded black-and-white postcards at the back, with army uniforms and serious expressions.

'I thought we'd all go to the pub for lunch,' Great Grandma says to my wife, breaking the spell, 'by car.' She's clearly not keen on me pushing her there.

As I drive, with Great Grandma in the front passenger seat, I wonder about those photographs. The connections of love, the hidden stories.

We pull up in the pub car park. There is one other car. The children's play area is a single slide in need of repair. Walking into the pub I notice there are over 50 'specials' chalked up on the blackboard, rendering the meaning of the word special null and void. We take a table in the middle of the pub. Toby bangs his water bottle on the high chair for attention, Caleb flaps the menu at his face and Maisie-Joy muses over a Princess crossword puzzle.

We get talking about Great Grandma's childhood.

'Well, I wasn't raised by my mam and dad was I?' she tells us. 'After five months I was carted off to my grandma round the corner.' Hannah and I pose questions between the banging-flapping-scribbling noises of our children, our usual weekend soundtrack, and place our orders. The food is with us in minutes, suggesting it was ready before we arrived.

'My younger sister came along soon after I was born, so I was turfed out and then a brother, Thomas, came along. I never knew much about him. I lost my sister when she was nine, I'd just turned ten.' Great Grandma pauses, then cuts into her soft vegetables. There's nothing wrong with her memory.

There are moments like this when you learn some tiny fact about someone and it casts a new frame around your perception of them.

'What happened to your sister?' I ask.

She continues. 'She fell in a playground and cut her arm. It formed an abscess, which got worse on the inside and the blood-poisoning killed her. Soon after that my mam and dad parted. They couldn't cope with Maisie's death, I guess. Of course, no one talked about those things back then, did they? Mam went off into service and Dad just... went. Well, I never saw 'em again, did I?'

'Hang on,' I think, 'did she really just say Maisie?' Yes, she did. I wonder what it was like for Great Grandma just 6 years ago when our own daughter Maisie-Joy Beatrice was born. What was it like to have a great-granddaughter with the same name as the sister she lost? When we return to her bungalow she gets out her birth certificate. Then we see her mother's name: Beatrice. We didn't know any of this when we named our daughter.

We chose the name 'Maisie' as it was the Scottish form of Margaret, my mum's middle name. We liked the connection. The name 'Joy' indicated our attitude toward the future, putting sadness behind us. And Beatrice? That was just a name we plucked out of the baby-names book whilst washing up in the kitchen one evening because of its meaning: 'Bringer of Happiness'.

Does life reveal connections when it's ready? Are there invisible wires between all the photographs?

Pieces of our story can remain alive inside us, waiting for airtime, for a safe place. Like my dad telling the story of losing his older brother Graham, as we sat on the creaky mattress at my mum's bedside on the last day of her life. Perhaps too often we rehearse them over in our heads, letting them define us, becoming a conclusion we navigate our lives by. But life is always changing. Our story only makes sense in the light of the future, which isn't fixed.

Back in her overheated lounge, leaning forward in her chair, Great Grandma jots down on a scrap of paper all the details she can recall of her parents and family. The photographs look on, witnesses to her scribbling. My wife promises to do some research. To dig deeper.

Great Grandma still has unanswered questions about her life and the bulk of 91 years is a long time to carry them. How do people cope with being rejected, bereaved, and kept in the dark about it all? Seems like Great Grandma's approach is to not bury the questions.

Then she writes something that makes me laugh, after all these previously unknown connections about family names coming to light. Next to 'Place of birth' she writes 'Brighton Street'. Of all the street names in all the country. Brighton Street. Seems like talking to Great Grandma has unearthed something, like she was destined to be a part of this marathon journey with my uncle. Stars in the same constellation. A family who need each other, held together by stories across a century. It's just the encouragement I need as we head into two of the worst months of winter storms our country has seen for decades.

THE JOY OF WINTER

Endurance isn't just the ability to bear a hard thing, but to turn a hard thing into glory.

William Barclay

'Time for parkrun, kids!' I shout upstairs.

Bedroom doors creak open and they bound down two stairs at a time, so loud the neighbours can hear the thuds. Most children are possibly still in bed, but ours are in their running kit. My wife and I drag our running kit from the radiators, where it lives for most of winter. I put shorts on.

It takes 10 minutes to remove from the car the snow that lay neatly upon it like a duvet, then scrape the ice underneath which clings to the windows for comfort. Once we are all inside and belted up, I turn the engine on. The thermometer says 0.0 degrees, the zeroes looking like two surprised eyes, as if in protest at being woken up. We drive for 40 minutes through the snow. This is proper January weather.

We arrive at Newbold Comyn near Leamington Spa with a minute to spare before the parkrun starts, and huddle together at the back of nearly 200 runners. We listen to the course marshal's final instructions. That's when my internal voice of misery starts.

'Why have we driven all this way through the snow to do THIS?'

My kids bounce up and down on the spot, I grip the handles of Toby's pushchair. Give me the surplus warmth from Great Grandma's bungalow last week, please.

A whistle blasts. Everyone sprints off, leaving me pushing Toby in his three-wheeled buggy through slush at 0.1 miles per hour. Pushing the buggy has been a useful feature in my weekly training plan for 2 months now, getting me used to running with my arms out in front like I'm a zombie. A habit reinforced by going out on New Year's Day with my sister, who has had a foot operation and become a temporary wheelchair user. Strangely, her recovery accelerated after she had a taste of me freewheeling her down the steep hill from Broadway Tower, the highest castle in the Cotswolds.

'Why... am I... doing... th... th... this?' Half a dozen volunteers in bright yellow jackets cheer us on, happy at nine o'clock, confident we will be last back. Then I notice my daughter, running next to me, and between snowflakes that are falling like scraps of paper, I see her smiling.

'Running is a display of playfulness,' says philosopher Mark Rowlands. We notice it when children run. They remind us that running is more than obsessive clock-watching and teeth-clenching defiance as we lunge across a finish line. What do children do most easily when they run? They laugh. Like the two are twins, running and joy, hand in hand. Childhood and running, exploration and exuberance, are hard-wired in all of us. The sofa and stopwatch have so much to answer for.

We trudge through the first few fields, buggy wheels spinning in sludge, watching the other runners escape ahead. Some ladies near to us cheer my daughter on.

'You're doing well, sweetheart!' they shout. My daughter looks up at me, smiling, angel-like.

'Parkrun is for everyone, from beginners to Olympians,' say the people at parkrun HQ. In fact, they insist that parkrun is always written as one word and with a lower case 'p' to emphasise its inclusivity. It started with just 13 runners in Bushy Park, Teddington in 2004, the idea of Paul Sinton-Hewitt.

It was the only free weekly 5-km timed event in the UK, but by 2007, to cope with growing demand, other parkrun events in Wimbledon and Banstead Woods in Surrey kicked off. The phenomenon of parkrun is a community event, now happening all over the UK and spreading across the world faster than you can say 'Mo Farah'. It happens in hundreds of locations across England and involves well over half a million runners (joggers, buggy-pushers, etc.), including five Spriggses in shorts from a small Warwickshire village.

Sinton-Hewitt expected a couple of dozen club runners to like it. He didn't realise he was launching a global brand. Still it grows, appealing to those who want to give running a go, liberated from unforgiving tarmac, distanced from grumbling traffic, and released from the pressure of racing. All runs are timed and logged on the parkrun website via a swipe of your personal barcode, which means for me pushing Toby today my average position will plummet from a hard-earned ninth to something with three digits. Anything for the kids. But what do they think of it?

Next to my daughter's bedside is a purple notebook, in which for the last 2 years we've taken it in turns to write questions to each other, then answer.

'What do you enjoy about parkrun?' I wrote to her. She replied using a blunt pencil so all the letters were double thickness, as if for emphasis.

'Good queschun daddy. I enjoy doing the sprint at the end. I like running with you. And going to the cofee shop afterwoods.' I resisted the parental urge to correct her spelling.

Our daughter loves it, but I still wrestle with the same questions most parents would have in this scenario. Some would say we are being too pushy. Is 6 years of age too young to run 5 km (taking 35 minutes)? Are we setting her up for injury or failure? It comes down to two things. Firstly, we always give our children the choice – to run, watch or volunteer. Just not the option of a weekend lie-in, as they'll get plenty of those in the years to come. Secondly, it's about them leading the way. We encourage them to listen to how their body feels, and to not give up easily; like when our daughter fell over and grazed her knee, she learned something valuable that day about getting back up and keeping going to the end. If they want to go for a good run-time that is up to them, but that's not what parkrun is about. It's about the run, not the race; the taking part is what counts.

The parkrun team have thought about this. Marshalling as a volunteer gets you 'points' in the same way joining in and running does. We've noticed children love the chance to volunteer, not necessarily because of any reward, they just love cheering people on and pointing the way. In fact, truth be known, they love wearing oversized yellow marshalling vests.

Just before kilometre 2 there is a hill. We keep going until we see the radio masts through the bare branches. This is the only notable climb along the 5-km route but it whips the energy from your legs and lungs. And wheels, in our case. A marshal cheers us on, left arm pointing the way.

Every runner could consider giving something back through volunteering. Many do. Without volunteering, the fabric of shared running opportunities would disappear. For nearly a decade my uncle organised the Horsham 10-km race, bringing two of his passions together – his local running club (Horsham Joggers) and the Horsham Lions, a voluntary organisation which raises thousands of pounds for local causes each year. This is why, come marathon race day, Uncle Andrew has a cuddly toy lion with him.

'The chap who headed up the 10-km race was moving on, and I didn't want it to fall through,' he told me. 'So I said I'd take it on.'

This is no small thing: promoting an event, organising administration for over 400 runners – 'none of it was online when I was doing it!' my uncle says – recruiting marshals, delegating water stations, negotiating with Brooks as the race sponsor, getting race numbers out.

'They've just started doing chip-timing, but that adds a few quid per runner,' he said. Running and volunteering have a symbiotic relationship. If one only takes from it, then it ends up bankrupt. You have to put something in, and Uncle Andrew has been a great example of doing so.

As we turn into the field, where 100 metres away the temporary 'Finish' banner wobbles, I say the words my daughter has asked me to say at this point: 'On your marks, get set, go supersonic legs!' This is the cue for her to sprint.

She darts ahead, and it's an effort to keep up, pushing Toby in the buggy through churned white-brown mud, which spatters and spits. I'm sliding like I'm on a conveyer belt.

My wife and eldest son, who by now have finished their run, come back and run alongside us. The tiny crowd, reduced to four, clap and cheer and point at our daughter. The mud flies up the back of her white fleece. White. What were we thinking? But right now we don't care. We are yelling and cheering, this is her moment.

'You are doing it, girl!' It's a voice, a huge voice, not just words trapped inside my head, I want the whole field, nay, the whole world to hear.

'This is it!'

This mud-splattering, twig-snapping, snow-squelching moment. Running as play, right here, silencing my grumpy mood and knitting our family together. She finishes with a smile. Then she collects her token indicating her place, gets it swiped with her barcode and then puts on an extra sprint to the pavilion to get a biscuit.

The parkrun events become a regular part of my training during winter, a chance to stick my head above the lonely parapet and notice other people are out there too, whatever the weather. But I am not to know that this snow-white January morning would be the last time I'd run pushing Toby in his buggy; that several weeks later I'd get a fever and not be able to run for the next fortnight; that we'd have to cancel Uncle Andrew's next visit because of heavy snow; that my wife would have to make a 999 call for one of our children who also had a fever and fell unconscious, causing an emergency trip to Warwick Hospital. It suddenly feels like we've hit reverse on the whole thing. My mileage for January plummets to 54, but I am glad our family comes through the month in one piece.

I don't expect, when finally returning to parkrun the following month, to meet a man there who made me cry.

THE MAN IN THE RED JACKET

Life can only be understood backwards;
but it must be lived forwards.

Søren Kierkegaard

He has a red jacket on, the man who makes me cry, and his grey sideburns peek out from beneath a woolly hat, as if braving the cold.

'How d'you get on?' he asks after the run, sipping tea from a Styrofoam cup.

'Not fast! The buggy had a drawing pin in the front tyre,' I say. He had noticed at the start that Toby's buggy had been discarded, sitting lopsided by the pavilion. Perhaps the buggy had trauma issues after last month's encounter with the kerb. It had proved irreparable, but not wanting to miss the chance to join in, I teamed up with Hi-Viz Steve and we alternated carrying Toby around the 5-km course, passing him between us like a baton relay. We finished second to last in just over 40 minutes and with the longest arms in the world. Unlike generations of British sprinters, we didn't drop him on the way round.

'How about you?' I ask. Other runners weave through, shivering in the pavilion, in search of flapjack and tea. Conversations about the run steam from people's lips.

'Well,' he says, 'I got round. I have an arm injury, so I have days where I can't do anything. It was just good to be out there.'

Him, plus 228 others on a snowy February morning. It's incredible how popular parkrun is getting, given the atrocious weather. It seems more folk are wanting to experience the 'theatre of the wild', as author and ultra-marathoner Robin Harvie describes it.

As I leave the pavilion I unzip my running jacket. This is a strange thing to do, given I'm leaving the warmth and walking onto icing-sugared fields. Removing a layer. Why would I want to do that? I regroup with my wife and kids outside, all eating chocolate fingers.

He follows me out. Then stares. He smiles, then hesitates as if to walk away. But The Man in the Red Jacket, I discover, is not a man who walks away.

'Do you know anyone with it?' he asks, eyes fixed on my unzipped jacket.

I look down and realise I have my Motor Neurone Disease Association T-shirt on. I thought I'd give it a wear ahead of the practice race with my uncle, the Brighton Half Marathon the following week.

'Yes, my uncle has it,' I say.

The man nods. We walk together from the pavilion, across playing fields to the car park. As we walk, he tells me about his friend who recently died from MND. He started with the friend's death and worked backwards. Is this the way to consider the story of our lives – start with the end and make sense of it in reverse?

'I went to his house at three a.m. on a Friday night and took him to the toilet, then carried him back to bed. That was the last time I saw him. He died on the Saturday,' he says. 'When I visited him, I'd take these engineering problems, like car engine bits, and ask him: "So what do you think of this? What would you do?" It was, you know, to respect him and his engineering background. It was his mobility that was worsening, not his intelligence.'

Picture it: in the face of death, two men sat staring at disassembled parts of a car engine, trying to fix something that was broken.

'Could he still speak at the end?' I ask. This has been on my mind as Toby has been attempting his first words, while an inspiring man I know through Twitter, Eric Rivers, who is living with MND, has just lost his last trace of intelligible speech. As Eric wrote on his blog, his speech is 'packed away in my suitcase ready for my departure flight'. At least eight in every ten people with MND lose their voice before they die. Communication technology can be a huge help – Lightwriters and eye-trackers and smart tablets – but they don't remove the sometimes overwhelming sense of loss. Of theft.

'Yes, he could still speak,' The Man in the Red Jacket tells me, 'until the very night he died.'

He continues. 'Once I called the MND Association because he was out of medication. There was none left in the entire country. They put me in touch with the manufacturer. So I was on the phone to this medication company in Paris, trying in my best schoolboy French to get them to send my friend his medication.' He sounds as if he still can't quite believe what he had to do.

The Man in the Red Jacket is not a man who walks away.

Medication for MND is limited. Riluzole is the recommended drug for ALS (the form of MND my uncle has), as it has shown to slow progress of the disease (but only for a few months). Research is underway for new treatments and Australian scientists believe they have discovered how to potentially stunt the spread of the disease.

'MND is like a fire starting in one neuron and then spreading from cell to cell,' explains scientist Dr Justin Yerbury, who says the research represents a target for developing much-needed treatments.

My uncle wants to do what he can to help with medical research. Every other Wednesday morning a taxi pulls up outside his house and takes him to Sussex University Hospital in Brighton, where he takes part in clinical trials for new drugs.

'It's quite easy,' he tells me, 'I get collected by the taxi. Then I'm picked up from the hospital entrance by my nurse, Dan, and wheeled to the Clinical Investigation Research Unit. I have a drip and I sit in a chair and read my magazine.'

I stand in the icy puddles of the car park and tell The Man in the Red Jacket about my uncle.

'He was a marathon runner,' I say. I explain about our Brighton Marathon plan. He smiles as my story spills out.

'Let me know what I can do for you. I mean that sincerely, for you and your uncle. I run marathons too, I did London ten years in a row, I'll do it again for my seventieth.'

My jacket flaps in the breeze whilst I am being undone by his kindness. Only later would I find out that my uncle also ran London 10 years in a row.

'When's your seventieth?' I ask.

'Five years yet! Anyway, I won't see you for two months. I'm back about the same time you'll be racing with your uncle. I'm off to the Himalayas next week for my birthday,' he says. From the metaphorical mountain range of caring for a close friend with MND, to the actual one of the Himalayas.

'Have a great time, and thank you,' I say.

He grips my hand. It's a strong grip, an infusion of strength for the journey ahead. The rest of my family clamber into the car while I lift the punctured pushchair into the car boot. It sits there, collapsed, immobile. I place my hands on the wheel as if somehow my strong grip could fix something that is broken. Tiny specks of snow twirl in the air. Tears fill my eyes, pausing, wanting to escape. Tragedy, running, connections. I don't know if I can hold it all together.

Brighton, we are getting closer. But before we get there I have to try and track down the most elusive man in the country.

TOM THE BLACKSMITH

He who allows his day to pass by without practising generosity is like a blacksmith's bellows. He breathes, but does not live.

Proverb

Tom lives at the end of a bumpy drive, off a nameless country road, after a hill with a gradient like Alpe d'Huez. He is not a man you come looking for when the roads are icy, but I'm told he's the guy for the job.

'He made a special contraption for my seven-foot husband pushing our son's pram so he's not bent over double,' my friend Jess had told me. The invention of a bespoke handlebar like you find on a bicycle was Jess's idea. 'Our blacksmith is just down the road from us, I'll ask him,' she had said.

Three months after Jess's novel idea, and countless unanswered calls, I'm finally driving down his jagged-stony drive with my uncle's wheelchair rattling in the back. I left the wet, green scenery of Warwickshire as dusk fell, at the end of my working day, and arrived in several inches of Oxfordshire snow. From green to white, like travelling from the Emerald City to Narnia, where it was always winter, never Christmas. An incredible contrast, given just 20 miles travelled.

Tom is a blacksmith and his workshop is an altar to the 1970s. Rows of bolts and clasps, next to hinges and rods, nails and screws – arranged in gold, silver and bronze like a medal podium. I suspect, with his sideways profile and distinguished beard-length, Tom may occasionally double up as Santa when the season comes around. He certainly exhibits the kind of joviality and friendly nature one would expect. I feel like I've come behind the scenes of the film *Miracle on 34th Street*. It's taken weeks to arrange this meeting because Tom is a man with no mobile phone, no email, no fax, no social-media connections and no answerphone. It's pure luck he wandered past his telephone in the workshop on my fourteenth attempt at calling. During this time Tom acquired mythical status, my Wizard of Oz, my Aslan.

I push the wheelchair into Tom's workshop for his expert assessment. I have it on loan for this purpose. The big question is, can he make it ready for a marathon? Tom scratches his beard as if the answer is in there somewhere. I'd hoped for a bespoke handlebar to be invented and ready for our practice race, the Brighton Half Marathon, which is in just 3 days. But any changes won't be made in time. We will have to race the half marathon without any adaptations. Instead, Tom has 2 months to conjure up something before marathon day.

'Hmmm, there's not much room at the back,' Tom says, sketching something on a scrap piece of paper, using a pencil sharpened with a penknife. I look around his retro workshop. This guy can fix anything. He certainly has previous. He is the blacksmith to the horse that will win the Cheltenham Gold Cup in a few weeks' time. OK, that's not previous. He also has a future, and not just as Father Christmas.

I can't leave the wheelchair with him. I need to take it to my uncle's this weekend for our half-marathon practice race. It becomes like a game of Memory.

'Here's the wheelchair, Tom, remember what you can,' and then – whoosh – 'I'm taking it away.' He has copies of blurred photos of the wheelchair from various angles, as if it was modelling for a magazine, emailed by my uncle weeks ago, which I had passed to Jess, who had brought them to Tom. In person.

Tom pushes numbers on a large calculator, like something out of *Honey, I Shrunk the Kids*, and talks in dimensions I don't understand. Then he points out problems I hadn't foreseen, such as how my uncle's head will get in the way if we have a crossbar handle behind it. New problem: what can we do about relocating my uncle's head?

'I've got to go,' he says, placing the sketches on the wooden bench as carefully as a waiter serving dinner.

Tom has hung around longer than usual to meet me at the end of our working days, but now has to look after his elderly mum, who recently came out of hospital. 'I need to get her dinner,' he tells me.

We talk a little more, enough for me to update my perception from Tom-the-Fixer to Tom-the-Devoted-Son. I leave his workshop and walk out into the night. The snow has thickened across the yard like an unruffled rug. I plough a course with the chair through it. The sky is clear, stars sparkling as if fixed in place with luminescent nuts and bolts by Tom himself.

It's a strange journey home pondering the loose ends I have little control over. I hope Tom will be able to invent something for us in time for the main event, now we are counting down the weeks. The night presses in, the glare of the moon reflecting off the snow like a torch. I keep the radio off. I like the silence, the chance to think. I notice the snow receding at the roadside, until it becomes a retreating memory in my rear-view mirror. I'm coming back to reality. The hard work is still ahead, with our first wheelchair race just days away.

BRIGHTON ROCKS

It's a great life if you don't weaken.

John Buchan

Motor neurone disease is a devastating illness. It's crucial to bank some good days along the way. For us, the half-marathon race in mid February proves to be one of them. But first I need to explain how I came to be stuck halfway up a children's slide in a yoga position.

Getting a place in the Brighton Half Marathon had looked precarious for a few months, not because of bad weather, but because my uncle's illness clashed with the entry rules established for over two decades. The other issue was the race had sold out a week before we had a shot at entering. All 9,000 places.

The race grows in popularity every year, so I knew I had to be quick off the mark to get in. I had made enquiries before it sold out, but the emails and phone calls rolled on for weeks. Time ran out. The race was full.

'Only elite wheelchairs are allowed,' event manager Paul Bond had informed me on the phone, so when I confessed my uncle's chair was 'from the NHS' there was an awkward silence. No room and the wrong type of chair. It didn't look great.

I paced around the garden, heart rate rising, my ear getting hotter with the phone pressed against it, as Paul listed objections. Risk assessments were conducted, our running achievements examined, medical histories were discussed. It was clear Paul wanted to find a legitimate way to include us – a refreshing change to the normal health and safety brigade – but there were rules and reasons why people don't do the kind of thing we wanted to do.

We discussed the issues my uncle's illness presented for a race of this magnitude. Predicting what his mobility would be like months in advance was tricky, and managing a wheelchair amongst a massive onslaught of moving runners when I'd never done it before was also concerning. It was another reality check. I got myself ready for disappointment.

We weren't planning on fun-running. We weren't after a Nice Day Out in Brighton. This would be a race against time in the most vital sense, and the best preparation we could hope for before the full Brighton Marathon in April.

'The truth is, we don't know if we'll ever get this chance again,' I said.

Paul considered it all thoroughly. I imagined him reclining, steepling his fingers, pondering our fate. Maybe with a patch over one eye. The signal on the phone was weak.

'You must understand Mr (crackle)...' I waved the phone in the air, no improvement, '... is a one-off... (crackle) is an exception not (crackle)...'

I ran up the other end of the garden, still no improvement. I climbed up the slide to get a better signal, in the manner I always tell my own children not to. It seemed to help. 'We will treat this as a trial and you must make that clear to others.'

I received this good news whilst performing a one-handed balancing pose on the slide, legs akimbo and head thrust forward. I was ecstatic, and immediately slipped down the slide, rubber shoes on plastic producing a rude noise of triumph. With the wind in my sails I emailed my uncle that evening to let him know our first race was booked.

The half-marathon course starts near Brighton's Palace Pier, then loops into the city centre, past the iconic Royal Pavilion, before stretching along the promenade – first out to the east, then turning back along the seafront until it reaches the Hove Lagoon. Then it turns for home. A turning point which includes some generously sized speed bumps, but the race overall is a mostly flat profile with maximum exposure to wind, tidal waves and gorgeous views out to sea. On a clear day you can spot King Neptune. On a foggy day I'd be lucky to see my uncle's head.

Being a reasonably flat course seemed a bonus, because when you're pushing a wheelchair you notice every incline. However, the out-and-back seafront course has two tight turning points. Paul had talked me through the congestion challenge in our first phone call: 'How will you avoid hitting other runners' ankles? Can your uncle get out of the wheelchair easily? Are you willing to start at the very back?'

Suggesting we start at the back stabbed at my finely tuned competitive spirit. I had pictured pushing my uncle along a vacant seafront, past an empty grandstand, discarded energy-drink bottles tumbling past us, seagulls barking eerily in the distance...

'Yes, starting at the back would be fine,' I said.

* * *

To help wake myself on race day I stick my head out of my uncle's downstairs bathroom window. It is 5.40 a.m. and a freezing fog has tethered itself to the rooftops. It is like sticking my head in a fridge. Still, the birds sing; they know it's race day. I breathe it all in. Uncle Andrew is in the kitchen, doing everything for breakfast one-handed, still able to walk without a stick, albeit a little unsteady.

As we leave the house, the fog gives way to an incredible dawn, revealing the splendour of the Sussex Downs. Then the day just gets better, and brighter, like going from black-and-white telly to full-colour HD. The day turns into a gift.

In fact, we don't start at the back. Instead, all 9,000 runners are positioned behind us, including the elite men and ladies, with their peculiar warm-up routines. Even the lady I embarrass by walking into the Portaloo while she is using it, next to the starting gantry, is behind us. Local TV captures me striding across the start line doing high-knee kicks, not dissimilar to Basil Fawlty's famous walk. My uncle's head roars back with laughter.

A few days before the race Paul Bond had got in touch again to say it would be safer to put Uncle Andrew, the wheelchair and myself at the very front, and have a 30-second head start. I suspect it won't be enough for us to hold on to the lead for all 13.1 miles, but for a tiny snatch of time a man wearing leggings and weightlifting gloves pushing a gent with a blanket over his knees and an air horn in hand are winning the Brighton Half Marathon. That doesn't happen in many races.

We swerve around the potholes by Brighton Pavilion and smile at those overtaking us. I point out some chaps running all in pink.

'This is Brighton, remember!' my uncle shouts over his shoulder.

We start up Marine Parade, a hill that goes on for the best part of 2 miles, the main incline of the race. I put my head down and hope all those training runs with Dennis, MicknPhil, Toby, my sister, and Great Grandma have deposited some strength in my legs. Runners pat me so hard on the back as they pass I choke a few times, spluttering water on my uncle's neck. The encouragement is immense. Soon we are at Rottingdean, 4 miles in, and turning the corner to come back downhill towards the Palace Pier. My uncle blares his air horn to warn runners in front of us they are about to be undertaken by a man dressed for the Arctic, seated in an NHS wheelchair with no brakes.

The wheelchair starts to pull away, my arms lengthening, like a magnet attracted elsewhere. The crowds start to swell, their noise peaking like waves, excitement frothing and hands crashing against drums, railings, bells. We sail through on an ocean of adrenalin. We see our families, their cameras angled, our names being called out like we are in trouble. We are in top gear. The zone. Flow. Basically, we are out of control.

I start shouting to the crowd about signing the MND Charter. I'm not sure if anyone is listening, but we are both wearing our MND Association T-shirts and I don't want this chance to pass by unnoticed.

The Charter is a simple five-point plan to help people see and understand what good diagnosis, care, treatment and support looks like for people with motor neurone disease. It has attracted high-profile support, including Professor Stephen Hawking and TV presenters Zoe Ball and Charlotte Hawkins.

'Many people with the illness die without having the right care, not having a suitable wheelchair, and not having the support to communicate,' says MND campaigner Liam Dwyer, who lives with the illness. 'We have got to set a standard so people like us are listened to and treated with the respect and dignity we deserve. We've got to stop the ignorance surrounding this disease and make sure that when a patient is first diagnosed with MND, they have access to good, coordinated care and services.'

Liam's passion rubs off. He recently crossed paths with the Prime Minister and got his message across. This took courage, as the illness affects Liam's speech and those close to him find it increasingly hard to understand what he's saying. The PM stopped and listened.

'One week waiting for an assessment or a piece of equipment is like a year in the lives of those with MND. They're essential to help us live as normal a life as possible and die with dignity,' says Liam. Liam is part of the same MND local support group as my uncle, and has helped the Charter get awareness in important places.

'His energy and determination are phenomenal,' my uncle has told me. 'He's even helping improve the design of wheelchairs so they're more adaptable, as every person is unique.'

Having finished my impromptu speech-on-the-run at 8.5-minutes-per-mile pace, we round the lagoon and over the speed bumps, my uncle semi-launching into the air. He is only prevented from being released into the stratosphere by his seatbelt. Then we see the beach, and the detritus discarded at the tideline, like leftovers at a party when everyone's left in a hurry. Some of the litter is on the course. The route is narrow and runners clutter the seafront, earphones in, blissfully unaware of what is about to happen. I lean forward and exhale with such intent, as if trying to turn the tide. Then I go for it. Waves surge and pebbles rattle like a crowd in applause. We dodge runners, left then right, zigzagging our way through, my uncle announcing our arrival: 'Runners coming through!' We finish with a flourish, helped by the cheers and smiles of Brighton's crowds. Our first half-marathon race is done, in 2 hours, 0 minutes, 59 seconds. By far our longest training run with a wheelchair. The noisiest. The speediest. The scariest.

Having crossed the line, we receive our medals. Uncle Andrew slowly rises and hugs me, and all his weight surges through me. After dozens of photos to satisfy the family, my uncle sits back in the wheelchair. The sea wrestles its way up the shore behind him. Seagulls swoop. I watch as he tugs at his shoelace, his grip weaker than he would like. There are gentle grunts of frustration, and so, for the first time, I find myself helping him get changed, tacitly. He doesn't seem to mind. We are a team.

At lunchtime our families gather back at my uncle's house over a post-race beef bourguignon, courtesy of Auntie Sandra. Our medals clunk against the dining table each time we reach for more vegetables. We get talking about the race.

'What would you do differently from today ahead of the marathon?' asks my dad.

'Well, I won't bother with my battery-operated electric socks,' my uncle says. The intention of these had been to keep his feet warm while sitting still for so long, but they proved to be overrated and underheated. I pause, carrots on my fork.

'I need to work on my upper-body strength. The camber of the road was tricky at times, I was twisting my body a lot to not lose control,' I say.

Then Elizabeth (my dad's wife) asks what sort of distances I will have to do to be ready for the marathon in 8 weeks' time. We get chatting about the Grand Marathon Plan, which is fascinating for the person whose plan it is, but not for anyone else. Several long runs of 16–22 miles are now scheduled (since my struggle in London, I've always aimed for my top five long runs to equate to 100 miles); a local half-marathon race (the Scorpion Run) without a wheelchair or occupying uncle to give my legs some speed; and then a 12-hour, non-stop relay run with my wife, called the 'Lightning Run'. The intention of this is to clock up 30–36 miles each, but in intervals, between dawn and dusk. All good stamina-building stuff. I could explain the colour-coding on my spreadsheet on my fridge at home, the difference between F for fartleks (sprinting spontaneously for short bursts, e.g. between two lampposts) and P for progressions (starting slow, then each mile getting faster). I stick to the headlines: 'Long runs, Elizabeth. Long runs.'

My wife, Hannah, chips in. 'What did you find inspiring today?' I finish my mouthful then respond.

'It was a great team effort, we were totally in it together. Me pushing, Uncle Andrew bellowing at people to get out of our way, honking his air horn.' I also feel inspired that, on my cousin Jo's initiative, celebrity runner Nell McAndrew and Olympian Jo Pavey were tweeting about our run. It was like the fog on MND lifted, the tide turned, if just for one day.

'What concerns you about the marathon, having raced today?' asks Jo.

I sit and think. I do have concerns; most of them are variables outside my control. I reflect on some of the previous marathons I've done. At my first in London the weather went heat-crazy and I fainted at the finish, ending up with a saline drip in a St John Ambulance tent; at my second in Dublin I cut my knee on a nail sticking out from the bed frame and then hit my head on the wardrobe door as I left the hotel to go to the start line (but I still got my PB down from 4 hours 8 minutes to 3 hours 29 minutes in one Guinness-inspired swoop); at my third marathon in Guernsey I had food poisoning the night before the race, bodily mess erupting from both ends for the entire night. I didn't sleep a minute. Nor did my wife, and it was her first marathon. She didn't thank me. She advised me to drink my recovery drink on the start line, which helped. Incredibly, we finished the race together in the athletics stadium, in 3 hours 59 minutes 49 seconds. Then I dragged myself off to hide behind an ambulance and resumed where I'd left off the night before, decorating Guernsey flowerbeds with recycled dinner. Our romantic meal out that night finished with me slumped on the table, the restaurant owner looking concerned about his menu. I shouldn't have run that day, but I had no stop button. Brighton will be my eighth marathon but each race, as I think about it now with Jo's question, has thrown up something. Actually, given my Guernsey experience, that's not the appropriate way to describe it.

Allegedly, when faced with a challenge, Winston Churchill said he wrote two lists. 'A list of what I can control, and a list of what I can't.' Having taken action on all the items he thought he could control, he said there was only one thing left to do. 'Go to sleep.' This is written in my black book somewhere, except I seem to have mislaid it.

I sit and imagine items separated on a list in my mind, placed under 'Control' or 'Can't Control'. Things like being ready physically, practically and psychologically are all within my reach. They go on the left. But dodgy mid-April weather, other runners' behaviours on the day, transport links, rebellious wardrobe doors, food poisoning, heatwaves, nuclear war, all that stuff I'm not in control of. That goes on the right. It creates clarity when it's all put together like that in list form. However, I intend to keep learning what I can, while I can. Learning. That's the official strategy, alongside another 300 miles of training in the final 8 weeks. The unofficial strategy includes red wine, copious amounts of Fairtrade chocolate and playing Doodle Jump on my phone until bedtime.

Auntie Sandra, having been busy serving lunch, is speaking now. It's one of those head-of-the-table speeches where forks are suspended midway to mouths, like Breaking News.

'It's been amazing, hasn't it?' she begins, 'Everyone has got stuck in and rallied round. I think because of who it is and what it is.' Then she talks us through what her kids have been doing.

'Sarah did a half marathon last week although she was poorly and raised hundreds of pounds for MND Association; Paul is training hard for the London Marathon and raising money for MNDA too. Jo is getting the quiz night organised, and it's proved so popular we've been turning teams away. Neighbours, work colleagues, Andrew's running club Horsham Joggers and mates from Horsham Lions. Everyone's involved.'

She pauses a moment as if running through her list of contacts. 'Yes, everyone. It's amazing. Right, anyone for more gravy?'

I recall that line at the end of *The Hobbit* when Gandalf the wizard points out to Bilbo Baggins, after all his splendid adventures in conquering Smaug the dragon, that he 'really is just a little person in a very big story after all'. Right here, as I eat my beef, I am that hobbit, finding my place in a story much bigger than myself.

Then Uncle Andrew reminds us he hasn't raced for 2 years, before today. His drastic decline in running performance during 2010 and early 2011 has been an indicator something wasn't right. Some would say running five marathons in 6 months, as he'd done, proves something isn't right with you in the first place. He ran at least a marathon every year for 17 years in a row, but that chain of finish lines is over.

'Well, I thought my racing days were over. I thought that was it, so yeah, I enjoyed today very much.' He looks down. I'm not sure if he's becoming emotional or just checking he hasn't spilt sauce down his Beachy Head Marathon sweatshirt. 'It was great,' he says at last. I know it's been an important day for him.

'You see, Chris, your idea in the middle of the night wasn't so mad after all,' says Auntie Sandra.

Her words jolt me back to that warm night and the suddenness of the idea that sliced my thoughts. My wife wraps up the post-race analysis at the dinner table by asking what we thought as soon as we crossed the finish line.

'GET OUT THE ****ING WAY, YOU STUPID WOMAN!' I say, re-enacting the moment. The language is a bit colourful for the Sunday dinner table, I admit. What happened was this: as we came in to the finish (completing our last mile in 7 minutes 56 seconds), a runner stopped right on the finish line in front of us to casually check the time on her watch. The finish-line photos show a sequence of images of us arriving at the finish, Uncle Andrew's face gradually contorting, his arms reaching out in stages to push the woman out of the way, the wheelchair tipping up as I try to avoid scooping her into Uncle Andrew's lap. There are things we can control, and then there are people who stop abruptly on the line as if they're the only person running.

What can we do differently for the marathon? Well, we can try and hold on to our 30-second lead next time, but it seems there will be more chance of us racing with a woman on my uncle's lap than doing that. Marathon day will bring its own surprises, and before then there are other lessons to learn.

STING IN THE TAIL

You learn the wisest lessons from your enemy. If you live.

Aleksandr Voinov

I stand in the kitchen finishing off a mug of coffee, and look at the calendar. It's the last Sunday in February. Not long now until Marathon Race Day. With our single practice race done, my training plan indicates I need to get another long run of 16 miles in. I have a local race booked in for the middle of March, the Blackminster Half Marathon, to give my legs a good speed workout, so I decide to do a recce of the course, as the route skirts the edge of our village.

I set off slowly, across the bridge, the River Avon pulsing, threatening to claim more of the village. I don't stretch before a run; a slow first mile is sufficient as a warm-up for the muscles. I turn towards the hamlet of Marlcliff and the rain is in my face, angled lines from a grey sky, stinging my skin as if being poked with dry spaghetti. On I run through village after village, the wind like a cold hand resisting me. I hope tracing the race route will increase my chances of finally cracking my half-marathon PB of 1 hour 30 minutes 0 seconds. If I can just take a second off that, I'll be content. The Blackminster Half is a recent addition to the race calendar, organised by Tempo Events, attracting around 300 runners, including many from neighbouring Worcestershire and Gloucestershire running clubs. I think it's important to support local races where you can. Not only do they cut down on travel time and accommodation costs, but you often discover new short cuts too for when the evening traffic is bad.

I turn right for another incline, shortening my stride and lifting my knees to keep the momentum. I've not seen another person outdoors; it's just me moving through persistent rain, on a road slicing through cabbage fields, earthy scent twisting in the air. The smell reminds me of school dinners. I sprint downhill, with longer strides and leaning forward to make the most of the gravity, past the Fish & Anchor pub, closed at seven on a Sunday morning. A heron parades by the river, a river now voluptuous, brown and fast. The heron rises awkwardly, like my grandpa used to from the sofa after a nap, yet is so slow and majestic in flight. (The heron, not my grandpa.) On I run, my face fizzing in the chilly air, and turn up Bennetts Hill. This long bending hill comes at mile 12 in the race, the last thing you want with a mile to go. It's known as the 'sting in the tail' and provides the race with its nickname, the Scorpion Run.

My usual race strategy is to go for a 'negative split', running the second half of the race quicker than the first. It helps prevent going too fast early on, and is a confidence boost for a sprint finish. That's tricky with a hill like this one, which will add nearly a minute to the race time. Sometimes in training

I run down steep hills backwards as it has less impact on my knees, a technique not compatible with chasing a PB.

It's a horrible day to train, but the coffee has helped warm my core temperature and the caffeine is a good kick-start to a run. The puddles on the road are so large I wonder if they've become permanent landmarks on an Ordnance Survey map. I stop going around them and instead listen to the splashing of my feet as they disturb the surface, and the sound of my breath. I feel beautifully present, and totally soaked.

I run through the hamlet of Blackminster, crossing the place where the race start line will be. I've still not seen another person out and about, when suddenly I'm confronted by four articulated lorries blockading most of the road along which I'm running, like they just can't be bothered to park. Each is from a different European country. I'm forced to slow right down and weave between them, like a needle through fabric. There's no sign of the drivers. I get through, feeling cross, but not sure which language to swear in. I don't want hold-ups, I want to get home. I turn up Blacksmiths Lane, triggering reminders of my visit to Tom the Blacksmith and wondering if we will ever get a wheelchair handlebar made in time. It's odd how a glimpse of something external – a road sign, a smell, a bird in flight – can trigger a memory. It's not so much gender, class, race or age that marks us out as different from each other, as the unique ways in which we think, react and respond to our environment. We create a one-time-only neural map. Our minds interacting with the landscape.

Rain causes my clothes to cling. My water bottle is empty, ironic in the rain, yet I still have 6 miles to go. I run past Long Lartin prison and consider myself an escapee of sorts, relishing the freedom of country roads.

My trainers squelch with each cold step and I regret not putting Vaseline on my nipples to guard against the chafing now felt with every stride. I grit my teeth. My knees hurt, but it's just lactate acid, a natural by-product of exercise. The faster you get, the more efficient the body becomes at processing it, thereby delaying its accumulation and extending your lactate threshold. The pain that stops you during a run is nerve pain, not muscle or bone pain. You know about nerve pain, as it feels like electric shocks. I'm now discovering how many nerves a nipple has.

I turn on to Buckle Street, the 4.5-mile undulating road back to my village. Still the lorries grunt and cars curse, some of them driving deliberately close to me. I thrust two furious fingers up at a lorry which swerves, forcing me to fall onto the verge into a hawthorn hedge. I am muddy and bloody and angry. I hope my gesture doesn't translate as 'please reverse back over my bleeding wet body'. It's not been a great run, but being run over by a 7.5-ton HGV isn't the best way to deal with it. With fury my pace quickens. I want to be home, safe and warm, with those blueberry pancakes my wife makes, in front of me.

Then I run one of the fastest miles of my life, dropping the tension from my shoulders, leaning forward from the hips and pumping my arms, making sure they move like pistons at my side. If arms cross in front of your body when you run they become a barrier, wasting energy and slowing you down.

'Arm speed governs leg speed,' the running experts say. I'm doing my best to only breathe in and out through my nose, in time with my steps, but it's hard to hold this pattern at maximum exertion. I lightly press my thumbs and index fingers together on each hand to make an 'O' shape, a technique Roger Bannister used to help him crack the 4-minute mile. The 'light touch' causes the tension in the hands and arms to disappear, the energy transferring to cadence, helping leg turnover to increase. Visions of catching up with the Scandinavian lorry fill my mind before I come to my senses, smelling the cabbage fields again, cresting the hill, and then down-down-down towards my village, and finally home.

I fall through the front door, 16 miles run: 'Every part of me... is... in... PAIN!' I announce. I peel off my white top, now bloodied with the memory of the run. My wife rushes from the kitchen to see what the noise is about. I keep stripping, not just my clothes but the layers of weather, the effort, the discomfort. I drop my running clothes in a saturated heap and within moments a puddle forms across the hallway. My teeth shiver. Immediately taking off sodden and sweaty clothes is part of my recovery routine, to protect the immune system as the body cools, but I usually have dry clothes at hand. Not today. My daughter arrives to see me standing on the doormat in just underwear.

She laughs and points, 'Ha ha ha! Look at your nipples!' They've been rubbed sore by a 2-hour run in icy rain. I have bald patches on my knees. Blisters on my heels.

The whole run was cold and uncomfortable, full of slippery verges and angry lorries, and the misted Cotswold hills, like a frame around my route. But somewhere in all that is a reason to get out from under the duvet. Running can shake awake tired bones, expose us to the elements, make us feel A-LIVE! It's a twisted sort of joy.

When the Scorpion Run comes round in mid March, I miss my half-marathon personal-best time again, this time by just 17 seconds (the following year I try again and miss it by 12 seconds). The whole experience is flushed away because the numbers aren't what I went for, like the wrong lottery ticket. Seventeen flipping seconds, equivalent to the distance of the final bend and home straight. Perhaps I needed a truck driver hunting me down for revenge. There will be other chances to express my competitive instinct, but for now it will need to be packed away. Sub-1-hour-30-minutes remains out of reach.

My training mileage increases from 141 miles in February to 160 miles in March. It's been mainly hill and cross-country running through winter, gradually replaced by increasing speed efforts in spring. Satisfaction outweighs the pain and outlives the boredom of being out on your own. My heart is charged. I feel dosed up. Joy comes when we least expect it, even in sub-zero temperatures. I just need to remember the lubricant next time and get back to wheelchair training.

'KEEP GOING,'
HE SAID

If you're going through hell, keep going.

Winston Churchill

He twitches the net curtains as I arrive for my next visit. I know it's Mick, because through the curtains I can make out his fluorescent yellow jacket. I reckon Mick sleeps in that jacket.

I'd promised to be on time because Phil has a medical appointment straight afterwards and this sneaky 4-miler has to be done before Mick's wife gets home. After all, Mick is still recovering from a lung operation to have a tumour removed. It's evident his recovery isn't complete, as he frequently has to slow to a walk during our outing, clutching his side to get his breath, moving like he's been shot.

'It's alright, Chris,' he says, face twisting, lifting his chin to the sun as if in prayer, 'I'll be OK, just... just... keep... you know... keep going.'

Mick and Phil both keep going as a rule. 'We do about sixty races a year,' Mick tells me as I push Phil in his wheelchair, turning out of his road and onto Bishopton Lane to face the early-evening traffic.

'So how do you do that when there are fifty-two weeks in the year?' My accountancy degree leads me down invigorating lines of questioning.

'Well, we don't do much in winter, then in summer we race on Saturday and Sunday, and you get midweek races too.' Mick says this as if racing three times a week is normal. I wonder if somewhere on Mick's body the words 'Keep Going' are tattooed, possibly on both feet.

Phil waves frantically as Mick hands him a plastic straw, which matches our hi-viz vests. We look like highway-maintenance men, wheeling a man along a busy road. In one sense, Phil can't communicate lucidly, given his cerebral palsy and sodium valproate syndrome, but he does communicate fun and he always puts me at ease. Understandably, Mick wasn't sure about me pushing Phil at first, as it's not often that someone else takes the handles.

'Sometimes in a race people offer to push 'cos they think it's easy to push a wheelchair while running. It's not. The grip and rhythm of pushing a wheelchair while running is very different. You get all out of sync,' Mick says. 'One race I was really struggling and this lady took over the pushing for me, can't remember the race now, but she was all over the bloody place, so I had to grab it back.' As Mick chats, between gasps, I find Phil's wheelchair misbehaves more than when I took Mick out in it before Christmas.

One mile in, a car approaches, at speed. I also hear a bus behind us. We are running along a narrow lane and there isn't room for all of us. The bus brakes, complaining under its own weight, shifting down gears, squealing in annoyance. The car forces its angry fender into the gap, regardless.

'Keep going,' says Mick, detecting my anxiety. At least I think that's what he says. The camber of the road is pronounced. I edge to the right to avoid the bully in the car and that's when I push Phil into a ditch.

I resist stopping my watch. I don't know why I'm timing our run given Mick's in recovery and we barely break 10-minute-mile pace, but my obsession with time is a habit. I try to pull the wheelchair back by yanking the handles. Phil's head jerks and the chair slides further into the sodden grass. I push, it just goes deeper into the mud, leaving its tyre-mark signature. I shake the chair, Phil's head wobbles. Then Mick reaches across and between us we finally get Phil back on the road. Literally.

The bus and car have long gone. It's a quiet evening in the countryside, the sun lowering its head in search of spring. Finches, kestrels and blackbirds get to see two men in suspect clothing, pushing a chap in a wheelchair chewing a plastic straw. Maybe that's why the birds sing, not because they have to, but because they – like us – are happy. They are doing what they can do, cheering us on, a riot of shrill crotchets and semi-quavers. Unrehearsed, but plump with joy.

'Keep going,' they sing, 'keep going.'

We return to Mick and Phil's home. By the sound of Mick's breathing he's in pain, whilst Phil shuffles in the wheelchair, reaching for a high-five. The light of the sun is no longer in the sky; it's in Phil's eyes. 'More! More!' they seem to shine. I put my hand on Phil's shoulder and say my goodbyes. As I walk back to the car I hear Mick's words ringing in my mind, 'Keep going.'

It's just a couple of weeks now until marathon day in Brighton. Training with Mick reminds me that mine is not a straightforward marathon-training programme, 500 miles from December to March. It's the usual hybrid of hills, distance runs and speed work, plus core-stability exercises (the truth is, that got reduced to balancing on one leg whilst cleaning my teeth), but with the extra spice of learning how to push the equivalent weight of a fully loaded shopping trolley for 5 hours. At full pelt. Fever and winter weather have impacted my mileage and runners know how vital an endurance base is. There are no short cuts to being ready for a marathon. If you haven't done the work in winter, then somewhere around 20 miles in the marathon you get found out. In winter, even 500 training miles doesn't guarantee you a good marathon time or experience, as my uncle found out in an early attempt at the London Marathon, in 1996. He'd raced four half marathons as preparation, all under 1 hour 40 minutes (sub-8-minute-mile pace), but by mile 7 of the actual marathon, just after the *Cutty Sark*, as the temperature soared his head dropped. 'It was after this the organisers introduced run-through showers,' he told me. 'I remember going along the Embankment that day and thinking: 'Why am I here? I am NEVER doing this again. There must be better ways to spend a Sunday afternoon.'

Clearly this wasn't the case, as the following year he rocked up again, having completed his winter training. Again. Marathon running is like childbirth, carrying its own version of amnesia in between the main events. 'Keep going,' our feet whisper, springing up from the asphalt. 'Keep going,' we hear in the escape of each breath.

'I decided I couldn't go out on a low note,' my uncle told me. A phrase echoing from that hot day in 1996 to today and why we are pursuing his last marathon together. We've crossed an invisible line. We are not turning back. No l ow notes.

As for his high note, that had come in Paris, where he achieved his all-time PB under surprising circumstances. The evening before the marathon, while crossing a road back to the hotel, Sandra put her foot down on a sloping kerb and fell.

'I encouraged her to get up, but she couldn't. Some passers-by called for help and soon after an ambulance arrived.'

From what my uncle told me, they didn't need GPS, they could locate Sandra by her screams. Then came the sirens and an ambulance ride over cobbled streets. A foreign hospital. A bleak waiting room. And the news she had broken her hip and that they would operate the following morning, during the marathon.

'Sandra said there was nothing I could do to help but run. No sooner was I asleep back at the hotel than my alarm went off at five forty-five and it was time to go and run 26.2 miles.'

He arrived at the start line, on the most famous avenue in the world, the Champs-Élysées.

'I was on target to beat four hours, but rather than coming undone like usual, I just got faster and faster, passing all the iconic sights,' he says, powered by the fact his wife was in surgery. He finished in 3 hours 45 minutes. 'But I crossed the line feeling gutted there was no one to meet me and share my happiness.'

Auntie Sandra remained in hospital for another week before returning home. But it didn't deter her enthusiasm to share in her husband's running adventures, having already suggested he enter the New York City Marathon to celebrate his sixtieth birthday later that year.

'We had three days of sightseeing before the race, and then the biggest pasta party I've ever been to,' my uncle told me. 'Something like fifteen thousand people. I remember arriving at the New York Public Library at four the next morning for a coach transfer to the start line on Staten Island. My mistake was I hadn't eaten enough before the race, because the queues for the pasta the night before had been too long. It was dark and cold, so I lay in a marquee, waiting for the start. Once the sun was up, the view from Verrazano Bridge across to Manhattan was incredible. That made the wait worthwhile. I ran well until mile eighteen and then the days of sightseeing and lack of pre-race food left me with nothing in my legs.'

He told me these stories in the pub after running the Shakespeare Marathon in 2009 in my hometown, where yet again he narrowly missed his intended 4-hour finish time, this time by 3 minutes. (One day he will look back and say this was his last decent road race before his legs started failing him.)

'Will you do this one again?' I had asked him.

'Oh no, I shouldn't think so,' he said, looking into his unfinished pint, as if his next PB was swimming around in there somewhere. 'There's still so many other races I want to do. In a few weeks I'm doing an off-road marathon along the South Downs Way, then after that a thirty-something-mile run near where I live called the Downland Trail.' Thirty-something miles? How is that possible? I had thought. Isn't the marathon the maximum? The ultimate? I wondered how anyone could run a distance so far they lose track of the actual measurement.

'There'll be about ninety of us, running fifteen miles from the village of Clapham mostly downhill to Newhaven, then fifteen miles back up. It's just north of Brighton, been going a while, I think,' he said. Given he did a marathon every month from spring to autumn, he didn't do any special training. 'I'll stick with my club runs on Tuesdays and Thursdays, a long run at the weekend, and just take the marathons as they come.'

When the Downland Trail race came around, Uncle Andrew struggled in the second half, tripping over badly on a chalk path and requiring help from St John Ambulance. He finished almost last in 6 hours 2 minutes.

My uncle had just unknowingly introduced me to the idea of ultra-marathons and the quest for running beyond measure.

'Keep going,' Mick had said. I remember when those words flooded my bloodstream, the day I took on my first ultra-marathon.

INVISIBLE LINES
OF CHALK

A sunrise is God's way of saying, 'Let's start again.'

Todd Stocker

Nearly 150 miles away Uncle Andrew would soon get up to go for his weekend long run, a habit of nearly two decades. He'd eat a cereal bar and just head out, maybe with some guys from the running club. A few weeks earlier he'd run the London Marathon for the thirteenth and final time.

At home I was creeping around in the darkness of my kitchen, getting ready for another race start line.

Digital numbers on the oven clock glowed green: 02:48. I'd had 4 hours' sleep, but that never seems to matter if I get decent sleep the previous night. I had toast and instant coffee. There was just one thing left to do. I began sun-creaming myself in the dark. Once lathered in UV-protection, I peered through the window, nose touching the pane, as if into a crystal ball fathoming the night, pondering what was to come. It would turn out to be the hottest day of the year, perfect for lying down with an iced cold drink, in the shade, all day. However, I would be lining up with a handful of strangers to run 50 miles in one day through the hilly outback of the English Cotswolds. To run beyond the measure of my limits.

The contrast couldn't have been greater. I was about to run the longest race of my life. My uncle was about to run the last race of his, unaware of the diagnosis that awaited in the near future.

In the week leading up to the ultra, Uncle Andrew emailed me. 'Good to hear you have the 50 miles fully sponsored. I'm sure after all your training and discipline you will complete the course in a good time and will be very proud of your achievement. I will be thinking of you BUT will not be wishing I was there with you!! My running,' he wrote, 'continues to be slow – mainly short runs enjoying the countryside.'

Getting ready for a race had become a familiar process. With each race there were new items to remember. For my first ever race, in Banbury, I had been ready in 5 minutes with shorts from a discount store, a cotton T-shirt and a plastic stopwatch. I had been keen and ill prepared. For this race I had creams to smear on, gadgets to strap on, paper to pin on, timing devices to Velcro on, and hi-viz gear to pull on. It was like a solo game of Twister.

I turned on my phone. A short text from my friend Tim appeared on the screen. I wiped the Vaseline off my hands onto my knee-high compression socks and read the message:

'And so here you are.'

Five simple words rested in my palm, chiming like Big Ben inside me. I muttered them to myself, over and over, the words gaining weight as they went deeper, percolating like coffee. We become resilient by turning the difficult events of our lives into stories. Is that what I was doing here? Were my feet trying to tell a story because I couldn't summon up the words? Storytelling makes absent things present, but can it do the opposite? Can it erase the past?

'And so here you are.' The words had my attention. But why? What was this really all about?

I stared through the window. The night was asleep; the window prevented me from disturbing its dreams. I considered my recent journey: after the five deaths in just over a year, including those of my mum and David, there had been my wife's headaches that had started as a dislike of bright lights and developed into meningitis.

'Phone 999!' she had shouted. I froze for a moment, then clasped the phone to my ear and made the call. I felt like I was falling into the unknown again. The Rapid Response paramedics came to the house, escorted her into the night, then into the ambulance. She was gone from me. My sister came and looked after our two children, so I could drive to the hospital. I put on the windscreen wipers but my tears were the obstruction. I prayed in half-finished sentences. I wanted results, change, peace, strength, anything that was going. By midnight Hannah was lying on a trolley bed in a room resembling a large boiler cupboard, her legs pulled up and chin tucked in, ready for a lumbar puncture. A hollow needle was pressed into her spinal canal and fluid removed, necessary for the tests. The doctors argued about whether it was the bacterial or viral form, so they went with the worst-case scenario, which meant another week in hospital to recover. I visited through the evenings of early spring, passing the blossom, but feeling dragged back into the stomach of winter. I left in the light, returned in the dark. We kept going. There wasn't a choice.

'And so here you are.' The past is gone.

A year later, as spring flourished once more, we had received every parent-to-be's unwanted news. Just as we thought our lives could start again, our very own springtime, Hannah phoned me from the hospital where she'd had the 12-week scan of our unborn baby. When the phone rang, an electronic invasion of noise, I just knew. My stomach knew. Her opening words: 'I'm sorry, I'm so sorry, Chris.'

'It's not your fault,' I said. So much said, in so few words. I carefully placed the phone back in its cradle, then stood in the lounge, hugging my two children, feeling like I should've been there with her. I cried into my children's hair, my shock smothered by the smell of children's shampoo and the knowledge that a new brother or sister had just disappeared off the radar of their lives. Warwick Hospital had become a black hole with no solid edge to grip on to and climb out of. Memories lingered there: my mum's treatment, my dad's hernia operation the week my mum died, David's treatment, Hannah's recovery from meningitis. Could someone please rub that place off the Monopoly board of our lives? We just wanted to use our Get Out Of Jail Free card, somebody please roll a double six. How far would I have to run to Pass Go?

That previous year, Hannah's operation was supposed to have lasted 45 minutes, but after 2 hours 30 minutes of waiting I became worried. I struck the bell on the Helpdesk to speak to someone, DINGDINGDINGGGG! My worry was marked out as a set of repeated footprints on the floor, fetching weak coffee from the machine, and back again to the waiting room. The plastic clock ticking... ticking... It had no heart. I listened to the nurse behind the desk, phone clenched into her neck: 'There was a complication, Mr Spriggs.' She explained to me what triple haemorrhage meant: 'Your wife has lost three pints of blood. She is weak,' she said, somehow managing to look down at me even though I was standing over her.

'My wife runs MARATHONS!' I wanted to scream, but my lips bore no courage. How dare she compare my wife to hospital coffee? Another dark night to get through. Hannah recovered in a room off the same corridor as when she had meningitis.

'And so here you are.'

But sometimes here is the last place we want to be. Finally, she came home. Finally, relief. Finally, decent coffee. To start again. It was somewhere in that darkness I knew I needed to go further than I'd ever gone before, to break the boundaries of my life.

'And so here you are.' To reclaim the present and tell a different story.

Is this the way we are formed through our lives? Layers like geological strata in a cliff face, different colours of rock telling our story, showing what has formed us and pressured us through each era of our life? 'That was the time when...' we might say. If we could see each other's stories, each other's losses, how differently would we relate to each other then? Our own layers are different to everyone else's, that's what makes people fascinating, but we all experience loss, a reminder we are all human. With loss, there is no Them and Us.

As I stared through the kitchen window into the darkness, I recalled something my mum wrote in a letter to our first son when he was just weeks old, for him to ponder when he was bigger. Words written at the hospice, in her final days before cancer stole her chance for any more letter writing.

'It is too painful for me to rush ahead,' she wrote, 'I must focus on the present moment.'

It sounded like something the Dalai Lama would say, but it was my mum, aged 59, hair lost in the battleground of chemotherapy. Dying creates clarity. With her life at its end she knew more fully than ever the importance of those words I was now looking at in my text message: 'And so here you are.'

Here is the only place we can ever be.

I squeezed the phone, and turned towards my front door. My wife helped our two children down the stairs and strapped them into the car. Lorries thundered ahead of us into the town centre, their heavy loads arguing with the camber of the road, sounding like metal pipes dropping. Noise never dies.

It's one of the reasons why I run, and am happiest running, mile after mile on my own. To escape the noise, and to tune into the rhythm of my feet on the earth. The jarring and jiggling of my internal state, thoughts seeking a safe place. It's like bringing order to the chaos of a child's bedroom, and every parent knows how satisfying that feels, however temporary. Running is physical and mental maintenance. Rarely do I feel in the mood for a run; the internal obstacles are familiar and faithful – stress, tiredness, forgetfulness, the elements, duvet warmth, a long to-do list. Yet I'm always glad I've conquered the apathy and clocked up a single mile, or many miles in one go. It all starts with a step, usually a mental one, and the knowledge I never regret stepping out the door. In the quietness of our everyday lives our decisions are made, and there on the run I can make some peace with my day, if not any sense. Training for the ultra-marathon gave me plenty of headspace.

My solo long runs at the weekend in the final 8 weeks of training had been like climbing a ladder: 26.2 miles, 28 miles, 31 miles, 34 miles, 36 miles, before tapering off to give my legs some rest. After the 36-miler, which took about 6 hours, 4 weeks before the race, I went to an engagement party for my dad and his partner, Elizabeth (they'd met a year before, then my dad proposed on the island of Lindisfarne under a rainbow). I grabbed a drink and said hello to everyone gathered in the garden marquee. Then I went into the house, lay down on the lounge carpet and fell asleep, waking 4 hours later as everyone was leaving.

I had also run two marathon races in a fortnight: the Paris Marathon, on my uncle's recommendation, where I saw the singing firemen, and then the Shakespeare Marathon in Stratford-upon-Avon, a year after my uncle's race there. It was down the home straight of the latter that I received an unexpected gift. My son, Caleb, nipped under the white barrier tape and ran onto the course, joining me to the finish. As we approached the finish-line gantry, we heard the race announcer loud and clear: 'RUNNER WITH NO NUMBER,' he said, an echo sounding above the crowd. Acknowledgement, not admonishment. Caleb has a photo on a shelf in his bedroom of this moment, the two of us, father and son running alongside each other, our steps mirroring each other perfectly as we sprint towards the finish. There is such joy on his face, as people the correct side of the barrier applaud and wonder what on earth he's doing. A runner with no number, but plenty of joy. It's one of the reasons I took on an ultra-marathon, to get beyond the numbers and into new possibilities.

Sometimes as a runner I get lost in data, inhaling numbers like oxygen. I've kept a running log of every single run since 1 January 2007. This is a confession, not a boast. I know how many runs I've completed every month, the day and time, duration, pace, terrain, perceived effort on a scale of 1–10, the weather, and how I felt. Every run is written down. I wonder, am I a slave to the numbers? It's not just the stopwatch and running journal where numbers can haunt us. The salary packet and bank statement. Waist size, calorie intake and bathroom scales. Exam results. Followers on Twitter. Numbers that mock us are everywhere. How can we escape them?

'Not everything that counts can be counted,' said Albert Einstein, 'and not everything that can be counted counts.' Life is like running and it counts, but not always in the way we think.

We drove 2 miles across town to my rendezvous point at Stratford Racecourse, where race organiser, Rory Coleman, was waiting. A needle-thin line of orange light sneaked onto the horizon. It was exciting to consider this moment had never existed before. All the mornings in the world were gone without return. All those dark nights too, forever gone. This was a brand new day.

It was 4.30 a.m. Five of us got into Rory's Mini, swollen hydration packs resting on our laps, energy gels bulging out of our pockets.

'Apparently you can get twenty-seven people in one of these things,' said Rory. By now it was light enough to see the lines on his face as he smirked. Rory got in the front with Jon, I was in the back with Graeme, Rin and Maureen. I'd never met any of them but we were all connected, our stories converging in a small car. My wife and children stood in their pyjamas and waved us off. I was thankful for the lift, even if I was packaged up on his back seat like a box of odds and ends destined for the tip.

Rory Coleman has run hundreds of these long races. London to Lisbon in one go, not because he missed his flight, but for the hell of it. London to Lisbon and 800 marathons besides. Running helped Rory escape a problem with cigarettes and being overweight.

'The difference between the mile and the marathon is the difference between burning your fingers with a match and being slowly roasted over hot coals,' says Hal Higdon, American running coach and still a runner in his eighties. If that's the case, then where would it put an all-in-one-go 50-mile run? We were about to be cooked on a scorching English summer day.

Driving down the A429 we compared our training programmes and nutrition for the race. Then Chatty Rin told us she started running because her other half was away a lot with the Royal Marines. Before she had stopped to think, she found herself phoning to book a place in the ultimate ultra-marathon, the Marathon des Sables, a 156-mile run through the Moroccan Sahara Desert, raced over 6 days. A race Rory told us he'd run ten times and coached many others to complete. Quiet Graeme nodded when asked if he had done one of these ultras before. A telling nod. Focused Maureen just stared out the window. How would the miles change us as we ran from one obscure village to another? How would our bodies cope running the near-equivalent of two marathons back to back, on a day when the mercury was groping for the sky?

Rory sped down the open road. The summer sky was brightening with each mile, like a fruit machine in its shades of cherry, tangerine and lemon. Not a winning combination for us that day. He parked on a grass verge. We spilled out of the car, then lined up in higgledy-piggledy fashion on a country lane in Farmington, in the middle of England. In the hours to come we would look vacant, tired and broken. But not just yet. The route would take us to Moreton-in-Marsh for the 20-mile checkpoint; then to Chipping Campden for mile 30; Alderminster for mile 40 and Stratford-upon-Avon racecourse for an unmarked finish line at 50 miles. There would be no grandstand finish or race announcer, just a wooden bench in the shade. We looked at each other and smiled, relieved we weren't alone.

It was 5.30 a.m. The sky was so clear it was like a car window that had been through a jet wash. I checked my GPS watch. It had a signal. I looked down. There was no start line marked on the road, so I imagined a scratched line of chalk at my feet on the tarmac which I was about to cross. A point of no return.

Rory called us to attention. 'OK guys, are you ready? I'm gonna count you down from five,' he said.

There was no big black digital clock with yellow numbers at the roadside, just a climbing sun that would be our enemy before long.

'Five…'

I panicked and fumbled for my piece of paper on which was a list, containing the reasons I was attempting this run.

'Four… Three…'

I could recite the list off by heart. I'd rehearsed the reasons in my head and out loud to the sky during my training runs over the past 6 months. Solo training runs, begun before dawn and finishing at midday, along empty roads where I would pretend to be a bird, flapping my arms in joy as I ran, or singing to the trees, from where the birds would sing back to me. They had their reasons to sing, I had mine to run. Now I needed my reasons written out in capital letters for when my brain melted, probably somewhere after the 30-mile mark. My reasons included the charity I was running for, HOPEHIV, who empower young people affected by HIV-AIDS across sub-Saharan Africa and for whom I'd raised £1,000 sponsorship. A reason to keep going is always stronger when it's not just about you.

'Two... ONE!' Rory said the last number loudly to make sure we didn't get stuck at the start.

'And so here you are.'

I took a deep breath. There were just 50 miles to go. But this was about more than numbers.

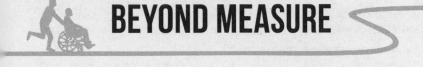

BEYOND MEASURE

*The measure of who we are is what
we do with what we have.*

Vince Lombardi

I stopped dead and swore at the sky. It was after ten o'clock in the morning, and I'd been running for nearly 5 hours.

Standing in a country lane, I looked behind, then ahead, consulting my map printout, personalised with rushed biro marks and comments about undulations and landmarks to look out for. This wasn't like the London Marathon. There were no marshals along the route, no advertising boards or balloon-crested mile markers. Not for 50 miles. We navigated our own way, helped by occasional stickers placed on fences by Rory a few days prior to the race.

I'd seen my wife and kids at the 20-mile checkpoint in Moreton-in-Marsh, with their 'Run Daddy Run!' banners, where I had changed into a fresh T-shirt and refilled both my bottle and hydration pack, a 2.5-litre bladder tucked into a backpack. It made the water taste like rubber, so I'd put blackcurrant squash in for taste. I'd had energy gels, rationed out at one per hour until my stomach got sick of them. I figured I must be getting close to the 30-mile marker, at Chipping Campden. My sister and her sons had promised to be there, and Rory had told us to expect a wobbly trestle table laden with malt loaf, fruitcake and bowls of wine gums. An incentive to get there and not be last, although not a patch on the checkpoints in the Marathon de Médoc my uncle had run a few months before this race.

'I had beer, cheese, oysters, ham, ice cream, wine...' my uncle told me, who ran the race through French vineyards dressed as a clown. 'Sandra bought me an orange wig, so I didn't look out of place.'

The 'Médoc' has a fancy-dress theme, which was 'circus' the year my uncle entered. You can picture the scene: a riot of clowns and acrobats, gladiators and animal performers gallivanting wildly through vineyards belonging to Chateau Rothschild and Chateau Latour. A dazzle of colour careering from left to right as wine-drinking pace took hold.

There would be no beer or wine waiting for me at the checkpoint, I knew that. But there would be bottles of cool water. Water! My hydration pack had been empty for miles. My lips were cracked. I had poured the last of my water on my palms and wrists (the radial artery points), to cool my core body temperature as the sun like an iron pressed its heat upon my head. An orange wig for protection would have been welcome. I knew I was dehydrated because when I licked my arm it tasted way too salty. I don't recommend doing this in public, it isn't a good look. My watch beeped to signal 30 miles but there was no sign of a checkpoint. My feet felt like they were sinking into the road. I was 100 per cent lost. There was only one thing for it, I needed to break that universal law for men and ask for directions.

A few moments later a young man drove towards me. I tried not to look lost, but he stopped and wound his window down.

'Need any 'elp, mate?' he asked.

'Do you know where I am?' I replied.

'Sure, ya near Chippin' Campden,' he said.

'Would you mind stepping out of your car, taking this hydration pack, and then pass me your keys?' That is what I was thinking but I held back the words. Instead, he gave me directions, and I realised I'd taken a road which rejoined a point earlier in the course. I got my bearings and retraced my steps to the junction where I got lost. I don't need to check my pace times to know the next mile was more suited to chasing a train along a platform than a 50-mile run in the heat of the day.

I finally reached the checkpoint, where my sister and her boys were waiting with a big sign saying 'Go uncle Chris!' I threw my water bottle at the ground in a burst of rage. Rory's girlfriend, Jen, was looking after the checkpoint and smiled at my fury. I felt silly, so I picked up the bottle and started eating cake. Jen is a world-record holder for running the entire length of Ireland, 345 miles from Malin Head in the north to Mizen Head in the south, in under 5 days. I'm sure she understood that things go wrong. Quiet Graeme and Focused Maureen were already there devouring fruitcake, so my detour had set me back from second to fourth position. Competitive Jon was already 46 minutes ahead, a phenomenal pace, over 90 seconds per mile faster than me. I collected hugs from my nephews, who had just received a lesson in how uncle Chris looks when he's Super Cross. Next time they'll add 'to the naughty step' after the word 'Go' on their banner. Replenished with cake and love, I set off, immediately encountering the biggest hill so far. It was nearly 2 miles long and the ascent was over 130 metres, so I walked, the blisters on my feet bulging like angry eyes.

'Make friends with pain and you will never be alone,' said Ken Chlouber, creator of the Leadville Trail 100-mile race in America. Friends with pain? We were joined at the hip.

There's a saying in ultra-marathon circles (it's quite a small circle, more of a dot really): 'Relentless Forward Progress'. Whatever you do, don't give up. The end is not yet. Walking meant I was still moving. To stand still would be stagnation. On and on, through fields with poppies in full bloom, along rocky farm tracks, through yellow-bricked villages, running as much as my body would allow. I stopped in the village of Ilmington to remove my T-shirt and let it dry from the sweat. I ran past fields of wheat, the surface looking like a sandy beach. Everything reminded me of a desert. I turned towards Alderminster, and realised I'd run 37 miles, which meant I was officially doing the longest run of my life. My legs and mind were in new territory. I needed to stay awake and on my feet but I was no longer sure what to think, which is where we really learn how to think. 'Ninety per cent of training for the race is in your head,' says John Foden, founder of the modern Spartathlon (which is run over 153 miles, from Athens to Sparta).

Running is a dynamic process for both body and mind. It's impossible to be the same person at the end as at the beginning. The universe is never still, its nature is movement. We are designed to flow with its rhythms and seasons, yielding to its invitation of ever onward, ever upward. Something changes in us with each step, each mile. New neural connections are formed as you push through the resistance of previous limitations. Micro-muscles are reconfigured as you accelerate down a hill. Fresh insights come up for air, noticing things you hadn't noticed before. We are always changing, from one version of brilliant to another, continually discovering what we're made of. When we embrace possibility, instead of resisting it, our lives spin on purpose. Thirty-seven miles. I'd come so far in search of this new territory, to rupture my limits and expose them as sham inventions of my mind. Every step now was success, even with 13 miles to go. Every step was success because every step gave me new feedback.

'How did you manage those last thirteen miles?' my dad asked after the race.

One might think of those last 13 to simply be equivalent to a half marathon. But I felt like I still had to run to the other side of the world. My secret for coping was something I learned at primary school: counting. I counted down in chunks of 20 steps, noticing each step from 20 to zero. Over and over again, a hypnotic rhythm, barely looking ahead more than a metre at a time. The idea of the finish line was banished from my mind. The mind can cope with the present moment; it's the future it has problems with. I knew the outcome I was going for, that was resolved before I began, but I had to lose myself to the process of getting there. Focusing on the contact of each step helped me to not rush ahead in my thoughts, but to return to a childlike state of absorption: '... too painful... to rush ahead... focus on the present moment.' Don't seek the next step. Become it.

Whatever is going on in my head seeps out in my running, I cannot separate the two. I am in my running and my running is in me. When difficulties are on my mind, they become woven into my neural pathways, carried in my bloodstream, revealed in my posture and stride. When our house sale fell through, for the second time, it was on the expected day of exchange. The moving lorry was booked. We were packed, but going nowhere. I was so furious I went for a run. It was better than screaming at the children. I ran for 1 hour, 2, 3, then 4 hours and still I ran. I kept going. I ran a marathon on my own in the countryside that day in search of perspective and the energy to fight again.

Several days later, I was still churned up by the loss – not just the loss of our savings, but the lost peace of mind, lost sleep, lost sense of control, lost sight of the future, lost timeframe – it was such a long list of loss that I went for a run again. I ran for an hour and kept going until it was another marathon in 4.5 hours. Two solo marathons in a week, but it wasn't the mileage that mattered, it was sorting stuff out in my mind. To change a mental outlook often requires changing physiology.

'If you want to work it out, walk it out,' the Romans used to say. Running and mental health are entwined. Running doesn't remove problems, but it creates distance, which in turn provides perspective. A chance to think again.

I couldn't change the unpredictable nature of the housing market, but I could change the way I reacted. I could loosen the way I interpreted events. I could stick with descriptions of events, not rush to conclusions that revolved around me, me, me. I realised I was too attached to the outcome of what I wanted and when, and wasn't trusting the process. I didn't know then our house sale would fall through five times. That our house move would take 5 years, accumulating over a hundred viewings. I didn't know then the process would cost us our life savings.

Sometimes even the light at the end of the tunnel seemed to have laced up its trainers and be running away.

'All will be well,' my colleague Mike would say to me in a quiet corner of the office, again and again, my head pressed in against his shoulder as if I was checking his brand of deodorant. 'Just one day at a time,' he'd say.

Mike was my calming influence. And eventually all was well. With much help from our families, my wife's persistence on the phone, and taking it one step at a time, we got through it and moved house. It was a miracle, just a damned messy one. That pain was new territory, but every step – the assertive phone calls, reconfiguring plans and budgets – provided feedback. A chance to start again with a new perspective, always more expanded than the last.

In my research for the ultra-marathon run-walking was consistently mentioned as a strategy to optimise energy conservation. At 38 miles, that's what I started to do. Run for a mile, walk for half a mile, then repeat, until my running reduced to a shuffle, my feet snogging the ground. I saw Quiet Graeme ahead. I snuck up and drew alongside him. We nodded at each other as I moved ahead in tiny steps. Third place was secure.

I thought not of the miles to go, but of making it to the next visible object – a hedge, a gate, a sheep. (The problem with using sheep was they trotted away, faster than I was running.) It's a mental trick I picked up from Dean Karnazes, the self-styled Mr Ultra-marathon, who ran 50 marathons in 50 days across the 50 contiguous states of America, and then back across the continent to get home again. 'There's nothing to it,' Dean says about such incredible feats of endurance. I think he's telling an outrageous lie, of course. It's not just your feet that are involved in running endless miles; your whole physical and mental being is in on the show. There's a whole lot of pain, but within pain there is always purpose, lurking somewhere. Dean inspires thousands every year to keep putting one foot in front of the other. 'Run if you can, walk if you have to, crawl if you must. Just don't give up,' he says. Make it to the next hedge, the next gate, the next sheep.

Thirty-nine miles done, I turned into a B-road with high hedges, and there he was, my dad with his camera, ready to capture my pain, frame by frame. I could barely lift my legs, let alone my head. I managed a grunt, like I'd regressed into the teenage version of myself. He snapped a few shots, jumped into his Peugeot, and drove off, not even offering me a lift. I saw him a mile later just before the next checkpoint. Snap-snap. Occasionally I heard him calling out 'Go on, Chris!' It was the only sound, his voice echoing through empty countryside like a penny dropping into a deep well. The sheep looked caged in behind a gate.

'Ha! Look at me!' I wanted to tell them. 'I'm a free man!' But, to be fair, the grass looked greener on their side.

I reached the village of Alderminster, and saw The Bell pub, then turned into New Road. A car was parked on the grass bank, its boot yawning open, crammed with large glass jars and bags of sweets and energy drinks. Still no oysters or wine though. Some guy had robbed the local sweet shop and I was so very thankful. This was the 40-mile checkpoint. My kids jumped up and down and galloped towards me. As I collapsed on the grass in slow motion, they piled on top of me. Everything ached, but their joy pushed back the frontier of my exhaustion. My wife refilled my hydration pack as I leant on the car and plunged my hands into the boot of sweets like the lucky dip at the summer fayre. By the time I needed to go, I wasn't ready. My wife and sister ran the first few hundred metres with me up New Road to get me going. I was anything but New.

'Forty down, only ten to go,' quipped my dad. Just. Ten. Miles. The race continued with a long steep incline, a 60-metre ascent. The sun was reaching its peak. I was destroyed.

My pace dropped to less than 5 miles per hour. Halfway up the hill my wife and sister turned and ran back to the checkpoint. I kept counting. Twenty, nineteen, eighteen... all the way to zero. Twenty, nineteen, eighteen... This is it, I told myself. Another mile beeped. My lips were stuck together. There was no willpower left to suckle on the hot plastic pipe of my hydration pack. The bag of cold salted potatoes stayed in my pocket, disintegrated, like my strength. I needed that sodium, those carbs, but I couldn't bear the thought of mashed potato when I wanted ice cream.

With 8 miles to go I saw Focused Maureen ahead in second position. I quickened my pace and started reeling her in. She was mine, all mine. Then Maureen stopped, throwing her kit to the side of the road and sorting it out as if packing for holiday. It was the slowest piece of overtaking in history as I shambled past, wondering if she'd set up a tent and camp chair, perhaps brew a cup of tea.

Three miles to go. I lifted each foot like I was on the moon, counting down from 20 to zero, then ten to zero, then five to zero, because there was no longer room for double figures in my head. Even the prospect of five steps seemed immense. My watch beeped. I'd reached 50 miles. Something was wrong – why was I not at the finish line? Anxiety rose, my stomach turned, but of course, I had been lost earlier, and I was about to find out by how much.

It's one of the things that causes worry and stress, not having a finish line. Not the literal absence of a ribbon stretched across the road to break through, but there being no end in sight with a problem or an illness. We survive roller coasters because we know they come to an end. We endure exams because we know the clock will signal time's up. We enjoy kissing because it doesn't last forever. Uncertainty reminds us we are not in control, but that's what makes possibility possible.

I turned into the back entrance of Stratford Racecourse. I knew the finish was looming. I could see the wooden bench as my feet ploughed through the long grass leaving two continuous lines behind me. My dad was waiting. My wife clapped.

'You've done it!' Rory said.

I'd just run the longest race of my life and there were three people to see me finish. I remained standing, in disbelief, my body expecting more. My wife pulled out a large bottle of water she'd kept in the shade and poured it over my head in one go. Rory dashed to the boot of his car and rummaged around to find a trophy. Somewhere in there was one with my name on.

That run of nearly 52 miles through Cotswold villages, with the sun making the houses look like butter, took me 9 hours 51 minutes. 'Just awesome!' my uncle wrote to me afterwards.

All five participants finished in one piece, on a day that fried our skin. But it also revealed a little more of what our bodies and minds were made of. I learned about trusting life one step at a time. I discovered something about endurance, converting it from a noun to an experience. It was no longer theory. It was in my bones, my brow, my toes. I'd made it my story.

The following lunchtime our family returned to The Bell pub, near to where the 40-mile checkpoint had been situated. The kids were sad to see the car with the sweets had gone. The pub was nearly empty when we arrived at midday.

'Hi guys, I'll be with you in a moment,' the barman said. 'Here, take this, it'll be your table number,' and he leaned across the bar and picked up a large pebble with a hand-painted number on. I took it from him and hobbled awkwardly to the pub garden, as if my legs were on back to front. I collapsed into a chair in the full glare of the sun and placed the pebble on the table. That's when I noticed the number painted on it. The number 50. I laughed so hard the cows in the adjacent field jumped in surprise. The coincidence – 50 miles etched into my legs, 50 etched onto the pebble – a way of saying: 'And so here you are.'

The memory of this race becomes the psychological tipping point for believing I can push my uncle in his wheelchair in the marathon. If you can climb one mountain, you can climb many. And when you reach the top you want to have someone to share the view with.

THE SURPRISE
OF SPRING

*The best preparation for good work
tomorrow is to do good work today.*

Elbert Hubbard

My legs feel ready for Brighton in just a few weeks' time, but my head isn't. Not yet. Something's playing on my mind.

The wheelchair handlebar from Tom the Blacksmith hasn't materialised. Multiple phone calls have again yielded no response. Somewhere in rural Oxfordshire there is a man who holds the key to me not breaking my back in the marathon. Another metre-dumping of snow in March means it's possible he's snowed in.

* * *

The bonkers British weather delivers the coldest March since records began and therefore means the event my wife and I have earmarked as the pinnacle of our marathon training is cancelled.

The Lightning Run was going to be a 12-hour relay run in Catton Park, Staffordshire, individuals and teams completing laps along a trail route. Coming just 3 weeks before Brighton Marathon day for me (and 4 weeks before the London Marathon for my wife), would have been a wonderful crescendo for our training, a chance to run 30–36 miles each on a cross-country 6-mile loop. The cancellation is totally understandable and a slight relief once we'd seen the weather forecast. The thought of driving for over an hour on icy roads, then camping in snow, is not attractive.

The cancellation blows a massive hole in both our marathon-training programmes. But, given we have childcare arrangements in place, instead of loading up the car with a tent, stove and changes of kit, we both put on our hi-viz gear, step out the front door, and run together into a choking snow blizzard. For 3 hours we run through snow calf-deep in fields, being the first to disturb the immaculate surface, over stiles and along country lanes which look like the cover of a Christmas card. We are cloaked in white. With scarves around our faces we use hand gestures to communicate. The result is 20 miles together, producing a happy tick on the marathon-training plan. Thanks to the snow, we also have spanking clean grips on the soles of our trail-running shoes.

Race day approaches. My weekly mileage tumbles, tapering for the race in order to give my legs a breather and let muscles recover after 4 months of making non-stop demands on them.

Carbo-loading won't start until 3 days before race day, which will mean second helpings at breakfast, lunch and dinner. Eating cake will become a vital necessity.

I ask my uncle to say something on my blog about how he's feeling.

'My main thoughts leading up to race day,' he writes, 'are excitement at being involved in a big event again, and hoping for fine weather – that makes it so much better. I'm extremely grateful for all the effort Chris and Hannah have put into this idea; their drive and enthusiasm has been amazing and I continue to be amazed at what they are achieving. I am a little nervous, as sitting in a wheelchair for close to 5 hours is something I've never done before. Being pushed over the bumps can be unnerving and uncomfortable, but it's all for a good cause and my suffering is minuscule compared to Chris's effort in the marathon. The whole idea has brought our families closer together, which is a big plus. I'm looking forward to it. The champagne is on ice.'

In the days before every marathon I've run, I become extra-sensitised to how my body feels. Tight muscles, aching toes, knotted calves. After so many miles of training, everything starts hurting. I'm certainly not speechless about all this. The physical pain and mental fatigue leak out in verbal form, coupled with expansive hand gestures to illustrate the perceived enormity of my suffering, like fishermen describing the one that got away. Nobody ever trains for a marathon in secret. A kind of amnesia sets in about what you've done to prepare, even though your body has processed every morsel of effort you've given it to chew on.

It's getting serious now. Radio interviews about what we are attempting to do have me up at 5 a.m., and I have to make sure my voice is warmed up so I don't sound like gravel being raked. I sneak into the playroom and warm my voice up by singing through the alphabet, although at that time in the morning it's hard to remember the letters in the right order. We get messages of support from Esther at the MND Association and Clem at Martlets Hospice, the two charities for whom we are running. They retweet my blog and send messages with smiley-face icons in them. My uncle does interviews with his local papers. Then a cousin I've not had contact with for a decade makes a donation of £500, a significant leap towards our personal target of £2,620. I get a notification on my mobile just as I'm about to deliver a lesson on alcohol in a school, with inspectors in tow. I probably look deliriously drunk with glee; the donation has me welling up as I set up the equipment. The donation gets my adrenalin going and I deliver one of the finest presentations of my life.

'Wow, where did that come from?' my colleague remarks at the end. It's clear we're not in this alone, my uncle and I, but I feel like I'm running out of words to adequately express my gratitude.

Perhaps it's time to let my feet do the talking.

The week before the marathon my friend Jess arranges to meet me. In the back of her car is a deceptively simple and elegantly fashioned wheelchair handlebar crafted just for us by Tom the Blacksmith. A horizontal bar with handgrips and two long vertical rods with holes at their base to attach to the wheelchair frame. Laying it flat on the floor it looks like the mathematical symbol Pi. It's like all my Personal Best Times have come at once. The relief of finally having the handlebar is short-lived as Jess's brand new car breaks down in the middle of the car-park entrance. In the end, on her insistence, my family and I leave her to sort it out. Stuck, going nowhere fast. I hope it's not an omen for our race.

The final week includes a few short runs, nothing speedy, just keeping my legs ticking over. As the mileage plummets, my mind begins racing. The people I've met, the stories I've heard, the reality of what we're taking on. I've learned so much, not just about an illness, but about a mindset, the depth of human resolve and the quality of endurance. A quality that seems anachronistic. These days our culture has regressed to celebrating the 'instant': instant fame (talent shows); instant wealth (lottery); instant food (microwaves); instant love (online dating); instant coffee (well, you have to wait for the kettle to boil). I'm not saying all that is wrong; it's just the emphasis I question. Endurance is clearly not sexy.

One evening, worn out from running 51 miles in the week, I had lain on my sofa. It was so quiet I could hear the plugs humming. My head was stacked with questions: Why run over 500 miles through snow, rain and fog? Why research an illness I knew nothing about? Why the daily worry about whether we'll make it to the start line? What about the wheelchair? How will my uncle cope? What on earth am I doing? I wrote a poem on my blog to remind me of what this was all about.

The night before the race, I read it again.

'One day'

One day to run, one day to push,
One day to wave, cheer, feel the rush;
One day to enjoy the breeze on our skin, hear the
   crowd chanting, cheering us further on and further in;

Chanting and cheering: 'An-dy! An-dy!'
A sound to behold and soak in; absorb all the
  humanity, the hilarity and hope in.

One day to linger with the masses on the start line,
making new friends in fancy dress, and waiting for
  gun fire;
then move with the throng,
running in zigzags, and zooming along,
heaving and weaving through the crowd,
our families adding strength, their hearts cheering loud;
the smell of Deep Heat amid sweeping feet, our
  nerves in a mess, for this is 26.2 miles, we run for
  nothing less;
Feeling the urge to race, the surge of pace;
Andrew lift your chin, show your face;
You are not invisible, MND has not conquered you.

One day honed by months of desire, dedication and
  doing it, yes here we are running it, knowing that
  THIS IS IT! This day is on fire! It's here, at last we
  are here!

One day to remember all the races and the miles,
the history of a hobby that's raised money, raised
  hopes, raised smiles;
endurance and enjoyment;
a kind of employment;
flirting with capability, and Vaseline deployment;

One day to be proud, yes to be bloody proud, thank
you, because WE ARE in the race, living not dying,
did you hear us coming MND?
Chanting and cheering,
One day to silence you, let love of family ring loud
and true;
Chanting and cheering again, yes again, 'An-dy!
An-dy!'
You are not forgotten, MND has not conquered
you.

Today is one day not to just stand and shake a fist
at you MND, but to face you, make you known,
somehow make a gift of you;
to say to the sadness of this illness: 'though you are
unwelcome, yet we choose how to receive from
you, time that is precious and friendship made
new';
One day to whizz in an NHS wheelchair,
along Brighton's fair coast, salty sea-wind in our
hair;
Race like we're free of MND, a day we hope for in
a future history;
One day – Today – love overcomes fear;
Hope draws near;
Listen to the crowd cheer!
Uncle Andrew, we are HERE!

One day to be thankful again and again, for our
patient families who've come this far, waited this
long; felt our aches, shared our song;

One day to clock up a bag full of miles, and push
  for a finish line,
one last race, one final time;
A gentle reminder we all have a finish line we are
  moving towards...
Just a gentle reminder...

So today is one day, just one simple April day to live
  like it matters,
grit our teeth 'til the usual doubts shatter;
let muscles ache and blisters form;
let knee-pain rise, mental fears storm;
let the knowledge come forth that this day has
  meaning and memory,
it has promise and power,
it holds decision and destiny;
it tells not just one story but many MANY stories,
Somewhere in here is your story too,
Ask for it, look for it, it will be given to you.

You see the moving river of runners doing what
  they do?
We run because we can, we race because we must;
One day, Today
we are ready for you;
Brighton: Are you ready for us?

I close the blog and pack my things for race day.

TIGER IN PRESTON PARK

How absurd human beings are and how magnificent.

Benjamin Zander

You open your eyes. For a moment everything is normal. You breathe out. You take in the room in the half-light. Then the panic smacks you in the face: IT'S RACE DAY.

The first thing I felt was yesterday's exhaustion. The day before we'd driven 3 hours in the rain to my uncle's house, where Auntie Sandra's soup made the world feel a better place again. Then my family had tackled Brighton city centre to get to the Marathon Expo to collect our race numbers. I made sure I had my personal identity information as well as my uncle's, plus a signed letter from him authorising me to collect his race number. The trip would have been too much for him given his declining mobility. The envelope weighed heavily in my hand as he passed it to me, grasping the bannister for balance. Two passports, two printed emails from Brighton Marathon HQ, a signed letter. I kept those documents as close to me as Frodo Baggins did the ring. Although I wasn't going near the fires of Mordor, I did have to find somewhere to park in Brighton, which on a Saturday is probably worse.

Brighton had been heaving, the pavements drenched. The rain fell in unbroken lines, making it look like it was going upward from the road. Puddles lapped over our feet as we dragged the kids along. I should have worn flippers, which could be the next evolutionary step in the minimalist-running-shoe market, specifically designed for British weather. We entered the Brighton Centre, thriving with nervous runners, leaving trails like slugs. I visited the team of ladies from Martlets Hospice, who were tucked into a corner of the hall, and had our photo taken together. Olympic decathlete Dean Macey stood near us, looking 3 metres tall. Pangs of intimidation ricocheted through me. After a quick tour of the stalls in his shadow, I collected both our race packs. There was no queue. The less time on your feet the day before a marathon the better, so we decided to head back to my uncle's.

We arrived at the multi-storey car park, the sky still rinsing its hands, and sprinted up the concrete stairway to Level 7. For the second time in my life I got lost finding my way out of a car park. They say mental preparation is everything before a big race. My whole family were soaked, stressed, and shattered. We had to be up at five o'clock again the next morning. Frankly, the trip was the last thing I wanted or needed; the only positive was we didn't get ambushed by Orcs. And I did get the race packs.

'It's easy to become overwhelmed by doubt; a race can be lost before it begins,' said one of my running heroes, Charlie

Spedding, winner of the 1984 London Marathon. I idolised Charlie in my teenage years watching the event on television before our family headed off to church on a Sunday morning, when all I wanted was to sit and watch the race in full. 'Come on, get into the car,' my mum would yell from outside. The rest of us loitered in the lounge, television blaring, David Coleman our preferred preacher for the morning, all of us watching as much of the race as we could.

Charlie is the last British athlete to win a medal in the Olympic Marathon. He was diagnosed with non-Hodgkin B-cell lymphoma during 2010, and had 6 months of chemotherapy. The treatment really took it out of him, but a year later he was given the all-clear. I wonder to what extent Charlie drew on his years of pre-race mental preparation to help steer himself through such a tricky period of his life.

In the story of his running career, *From Last to First*, he talks about how, when a problem arose, he would deliberately switch things round in his head, so instead of reacting, he'd look for something 'positive and useful in it', he says.

What could possibly be 'positive and useful' about my family's miserable day out? I decided to treat the day-gone-wrong like a test, like when a performer stands on stage and tests the microphone: 'One-two, one-two.' You've got to be tested a bit to check you're wired and ready to perform. Back at my uncle's, with the rain tap-tapping on the guest-bedroom window, I sat on the bed and composed myself. That's when I saw the photograph. I reached out and held the frame. It was of my uncle finishing the London Marathon, right arm held aloft, the digital clock reading 4 hours 24 minutes. NutraSweet had been the race sponsor. I could not help but feel the poignancy of seeing his right arm raised like that, an arm whose strength has now visibly departed.

Before tea, my uncle and I had disappeared into his garage to attempt to put the handlebar on the wheelchair for the first time. We had clambered around the lawnmower, various tools and a stack of old bikes, and found a space at the garage entrance. A garage which within 2 years will have been converted into a dining room, and the old dining room into a ground-floor bedroom, when Uncle Andrew can no longer walk upstairs. With the garage door up, for more space and light, I assembled the wheelchair, rain thrusting itself across the threshold. My wife videoed us, probably wanting evidence of my attempts at DIY for the archives. My sister and her husband Graham arrived, darting from their car and ducking under the garage door. They hugged my uncle, then shot me a look of concern. Yes, it was me down there trying to fix something.

Several minutes later, I'd threaded multiple plastic tags through every available orifice – on the wheelchair, not my uncle. I invited him to take a seat, before explaining where the emergency exits were. Then we went sprinting in the rain, without coats, steaming up and down the road. I shook the wheelchair from side to side checking the handlebar would stay in place. My uncle remained in the chair, petrified, possibly with rearranged organs. I propelled us back into the garage, into the dry. There was nothing more we could do before race day apart from dry off and eat. After all the hassle acquiring the handlebar, it was a relief that it seemed to work, although 5 minutes in the rain wasn't quite the practice I'd hoped for.

The evening was lively, with extra family joining us, including my uncle's sister, Auntie Hilary. It was an out-of-the-blue visit, as if the gaps in our family were closing. Pasta and wine, photographs and conversation flowed at the dining table, full of interruptions and laughter. I excused myself and went to bed, but not before rearranging all my kit four times. A sort of feng shui for sportswear. The noise continued downstairs past midnight. I don't know when I found sleep.

* * *

My alarm is beeping. It is 5 a.m. One by one, family members stir, and breakfast things are placed on the table. I pace up and down the hallway, reading through my checklist, convinced something is missing. It's not desire; perhaps it's sanity. I stick my head out of my uncle's downstairs bathroom window, for old times' sake. The birds sound excited again, just as they had been before our last race together, the Brighton Half Marathon.

We load up his car with the wheelchair, handlebar and blankets. He's not wearing his electric socks this time. I realise as we pull away what I've forgotten. Breakfast. In all my fussing, I've not eaten anything. My wife comes to the rescue and thrusts a large tin of home-made cookies onto my lap. I eat the lot. We drive for an hour, leaving in the dark but arriving in Brighton in grey light.

We park up a hill and walk to the coach at the temporary Park and Ride stop. Auntie Sandra pushes my uncle and I consider whether she'd be up for a last-minute swap. The wheelchair has to go in the undercarriage of the coach. Just the wheelchair, not my uncle, causing brief separation anxiety. Then the coach takes us the short distance to Preston Park, from where the race will begin. Once the runners have flooded out of the coach, we find a space and start to get ready.

I take a deep breath. I can smell the cut grass. Yesterday's torrential rain has awakened it from hibernation.

We are here.

Early morning drizzle runs off my forehead and stings my eyes. I can't see. I blink. I see a tiger running towards us. I blink again. Yes, it really is a tiger, strapped to a man's back.

'Is it real, Daddy?' my daughter asks. She moves closer to me for safety. Now is not the time for an existential discussion, so I ignore her and wrap more gaffer tape around the frame of the wheelchair. The sound of peeling tape punctuates the conversation.

I'm losing my patience. Sticking gaffer tape on the wheelchair is proving a nuisance. I'm not a man with DIY skills, neither am I on good terms with gadgets and machinery. Once, whilst cutting my lawn, I broke our petrol lawnmower. So I borrowed our neighbour's electric one and broke that too. Having returned it with an apology, I walked to the next house up my street and borrowed their strimmer. Which I also broke. They were furious. I finished cutting my lawn with a pair of scissors on my hands and knees, which I'm proud to say all remained in excellent working order.

We are shielded by nervous crowds next to the Portaloos, which look like a spare set of Doctor Who TARDISes. I shake the wheelchair. I'm not convinced everything will stay in place for 5 hours or more. Uncle Andrew looks on, lost in thought. I unleash more tape. We are not aiming to be the first or the best. We are facing up to a life-limiting illness together. Running won't take away the disease. But can we rise above the sadness? Just for one day?

Preston Park is crammed with over 9,000 runners about to take on the city marathon, now in its fourth year. Self-styled as 'the London Marathon by the sea', popularity has caused it to become the second-biggest marathon in England. Today there are 7,000 barriers erected, 12,000 cones placed and 6 miles of branding. Nearly 400 charities are represented, from big charity names to tiny local charities tucked down a Brighton side street. Today's gathering will raise about £5 million, proof that even in times of austerity the Great British public still have a passion to make things better.

Not everyone is a fan of the modern city marathon, with its mass commercialisation and enough energy drinks to send a rocket to Mars. I understand that, but I still hear the heartbeat of this iconic endurance event, which draws so many back time and again. At the heart of the marathon is a quest to overcome, to say 'I Am Here', to give life a shake.

England cricketer Matt Prior, who grew up in Brighton, stands next to the rubber mats at the start line. He will officially declare the race underway in a few minutes, releasing runners who are currently poised as if in a catapult, ready to burst into stride en masse.

The route will start with a loop of the park, then take in the best of the city centre, including the iconic Brighton Pavilion. Then, heading east along the scenic coastal road, the runners will get panoramic views of the English Channel and glimpses of the glorious South Downs.

'Daddy, is the tiger reee-all?' My daughter is having a crisis. She stamps her foot.

'No, the tiger isn't real, darling,' I say. There's no hint of reassurance in my tone. I'm trying to get the gaffer tape to do as it's told without snarling and baring my teeth.

'Where are the plastic ties?' I ask, glancing up at my wife. She looks bewildered, lips tied tight like laces. She's less worried about the man-with-tiger warming up next to us and more concerned about my lack of preparation. She hands me the ties. Eventually they do the trick, four of them, plus a roll of gaffer tape. Hey presto! We're ready.

Uncle Andrew's daughter Jo takes photos, each moment catalogued for the future, when they will be looked upon within four sharp corners. Auntie Sandra stands like a bodyguard at his side. She's used to this. Without her faithful support over the years we wouldn't be here. We'd be in the dry, drinking cappuccinos with chocolate sprinkles on top, the chance passing us by. I wonder what's going through my uncle's mind as he surveys the park.

'Toughness is in the soul and spirit, not in the muscles,' Jo had reminded him earlier this week through her contribution on my blog, drawing inspiration from the Irish rugby team. His other children, Sarah and Paul, both said on the blog how inspirational their dad has been in how he has faced up to the illness so far.

My uncle eases himself into the wheelchair, a slight grimace as his full weight lands on the seat.

'Well, I never thought I'd get the chance to race again,' he says, looking around the park, as if peering through the runners to what lies beyond. Running 39 marathons (or longer) has defined his last two decades, since the sport found him in his early forties, overweight from too many hotel meals and office work. Today is one last taste of the running life. He takes it all in, like a performer at the end of a show before the curtain quietly falls. Then I hand him my bag of cold salted potatoes and energy drink.

I take hold of the handles and steer the wheelchair through bodies in various states of undress, through nervous laughter and conversations about safety pins. We warm up at the edge of the park with some quick sprints, to check everything doesn't wobble too much. A voice from a tannoy carries over our heads, bringing stillness to the gathering. My uncle and I join the back of the pack. That had to be agreed upon at the time of our entry to the race. Neither of us is used to starting at the back of a marathon. In all our solo attempts we've been hemmed in the middle, sharing armpit space and having toes trodden on. Now, we are in the green pen with fancy-dress runners and brave folk taking on calories as well as miles. There are runners here who together would fit every clothing size going. There is no correct body shape for participating, of course. Whether you're size 8 or 18, here not all the numbers matter. What matters is that You Are Here.

I crouch back down to twiddle the plastic tags and massage the gaffer tape, as if needing reassurance.

'Hello, Chris!' someone says. We are moments away from Matt Prior starting us off when Celia, an old school friend I haven't seen for 23 years appears the other side of the 2-metre-high perimeter fence. I turn in surprise. A long-lost hug isn't going to happen, so we mimic a reunion either side of the cage-like barrier. I introduce my uncle to Celia, whose husband is doing his first marathon. Celia offers to take a photo. It's important to catch these moments – to still the contents of a moving picture – so I pass my smartphone delicately through the cage. Alas, none of us remembers that mesh fencing doesn't create the kind of photo you want to hang on your wall. My uncle and I look like we are in prison, with a man dressed as a giant green telephone coming to the rescue in the background. Celia wishes us all the best and walks away. I put my phone away. It's cold, so I bounce on the spot.

As I jump, I see a pipeline of energised runners flinging themselves around the first bend of Preston Park, a mass of arms pumping vigorously, leaving their worries on the rubber mat. I hope Matt Prior isn't too overwhelmed by all the emotional junk being left on the start line, forever discarded like the end of a jumble sale, never to be collected or owned again. Will we ever budge? We move a few metres toward the start but there's a bottleneck ahead, and I don't mean the neck of the fancy-dress bottle of champagne. So many coloured vests stretch out before us, like the longest line of washing in the world. Horns and whistles blast constantly. It's a party in motion.

Gathering in Preston Park with all the other runners, in the drizzle, is about to turn into one of the most important days in our lives. I stand behind my uncle, my hands containing the wheelchair, like an extension containing all our reasons to run. I close my eyes and notice the rise, then the fall, of my chest. The rise, the fall. Taking it all in. Noticing my breath. Letting my mind be drawn into my body, and the ground rise up to my feet. This is where we are. It's a good place to be.

We inch closer towards the start line. I take hold of my uncle's left hand, the one with grip, and pray. I'm not scared or superstitious, just thankful.

'Help us enjoy each step, each mile, each moment.'

What's in store for us all? What will it take to refrain from leaving my uncle stranded at a bus stop halfway round?

As running legend Steve Cram says, 'You never quite know what will happen in the marathon until you're in it.' There's only one way to find out. Numbers 7687 and 7646, our time has come.

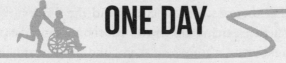

ONE DAY

Confine yourselves to the present moment.

Marcus Aurelius

The throng of runners creeps forward. I take a step. The wheelchair is in motion. It feels like we have come so far. My breathing quickens as we bump over the rubber mat, passing Matt Prior, activating the electronic timing chips attached to the back of our numbers. We are hemmed in, by bodies and noise.

We encounter our first incline just a few hundred metres into the race. Some runners start walking. I endeavour to keep the same momentum throughout the race, but it's early days and the mass of runners is so dense I have to slow down to 12-minute-mile pace. We are behind schedule. I take a deep breath.

'There is no schedule, remember. Relax the shoulders. Take in the crowd,' I say to myself. The crowd is thoroughly warmed up, waving flags and banners as if we were at mile 20. We pass the first mile marker and descend back down the far side of the park. I see other runners like us in lilac vests. Lilac is a popular colour for charities – it's unisex, inoffensive and goes with jeans. My mum would approve.

The only brakes on the wheelchair are the levers at the height of my uncle's hands, useless when going at speed. I feel apprehensive about how much concentration it takes to not only stay in control of the chair as it accelerates away on the downhill sections, but to also avoid the ankles of other runners. There are many ankles to avoid. It seems most people have brought at least two with them, so I need to stay alert.

Someone shouts at us. Above the constant bantering, there is a voice I recognise. Then I see him, my dad running alongside us, a camera nodding its lens against his chest. A memory is triggered.

My dad was a runner, a very keen one. But his knees won't let him run anymore. Back in his day there were no GPS watches, compression socks or pronation-control trainers. They didn't even know about hydration before a race; they just thought vomiting after a hard run was normal and necessary. A marker of true effort. Tough cookies, they were.

My memory is this: I am in our dining room as a child, clearing gravy-smeared dinner plates from the table, passing them through the hatch to my mum in the kitchen. It's unlikely to be the same day that Charlie Spedding conquered the London Marathon, but it's that era. I'm 10 years old. On the ledge of the hatch between the kitchen and dining room is a 7 x 5-inch frame. I get distracted from my chores and pick it up. It says 'National Record' on the gold plaque and I read four men's names engraved upon it, of which 'M. Spriggs' is one.

My dad ran for Sale Harriers Athletics Club and on 29 June 1965 was part of a record-breaking 4 x 1-mile relay team in a race held on the newly opened Longford Park, Stretford. Four runners completing 1 mile each, an event now archived along with cinder running tracks and the New Balance Trackster shoe. My dad once raced against Derek Ibbotson, the mile world-record holder in 1957. Derek was the Mo Farah of the 1950s.

'My dad. National hero.' They may or may not have been the words I thought in that moment, just before my mum told me to hurry up with the plates, but something germinated inside me, and it wasn't the dinner we'd eaten. Inspiration perhaps. Realisation that someone close to me had gone out into the big wide world and made an impression, with running spikes.

Somewhere along the family line, in a kind-of-accidental way, perhaps my dad's running ambitions became mine? A psychoanalyst would love to examine that. Is running a genetic obsession? Can it be caught as easily as measles? At the very least, I'm convinced enthusiasm is contagious.

We exit Preston Park onto a level road. My dad is still running, camera now in hand, snap-snap-snap, his bush hat bobbing with each step. He cheers us on. My dad is usually such a quiet man, but I guess that's what marathons do to you, or perhaps that's what the presence of motor neurone disease in the family does to you. It's not something to stay quiet about.

'Go Chris, Go Andrew!' he yells. His voice rings with emotion.

'See your running career isn't over, Dad!' I shout back.

I wonder what it's like for my dad, seeing his younger brother being pushed in a wheelchair by his son, in a race he's never had the chance to run. A dad who's already lost one brother, in that tragic air accident five decades ago. Do the years squeeze together at times like this? It's tempting for our minds to join events together like a dot-to-dot, and create some new meaning from them. The meaning we invent may not be accurate or useful of course, but as humans we're hungry for meaning. To make some sense of our lives. We want X to equal Y because that's neat and tidy, but life is way more haphazard than GCSE maths.

We head toward the city centre. The first mile is circuitous which affords us the pleasure of passing our families again, offering more high-fives, smiles and plenty of overused two-word boosts of support: 'Keep going!' 'Looking good!' 'Well done!'

Being cheered on is like a drug. Hearing your name being screamed out is a glorious adrenalin-boost and it's enough to keep you going for a few miles. If only you could bottle this feeling. I've made sure we both get maximum shout-outs by painstakingly attaching our names to the front and back of our vests with black insulation tape.

We pass Brighton Pavilion, one of the few landmarks on the course, accompanied by dozens of potholes. Then, as we approach mile 2, I want to stop. I want to stop and reverse several hundred metres, because I've just realised my friends Sam and Miriam, who I slowed down for, kissed hello and said goodbye to, aren't even supposed to be in Brighton. They live in London. What are they doing down here? It's a wonderful surprise, and it all turns out OK when I see them again in the city centre, leaving me to suspect they're running between parts of the course at twice the speed of my uncle and myself. We edge towards 10-minute-per-mile pace now the road has widened and the ribbon of runners is being unfurled and lengthened, step by step, like the unwrapping of a gift. I start telling my uncle about Sam and

Miriam, feeling emotional for the first time since we crossed the start line.

In 7 days' time Sam will run for the MND Association in his first ever marathon, in London. He hates running but a close friend of his, Ludo, in France, is grappling with the illness. Actually grappling is the wrong word. When I last spoke to Sam he described how Ludo could no longer hold any of his four children. Ludo was born in the same year as I was, and diagnosed at age 38. The last time I saw him was on Sam's wedding day, when we were both ushers in identical smart suits with red cravats, bearing identical happy grins, perhaps with identical aspirations of family life and parenthood. MND is no respecter of age, nationality, personality or aspiration.

We weave our way past runners, some of whom look aghast that they're being undertaken by a wheelchair. I wonder how Sam will get on next week. At this point I have no way of knowing that I will unexpectedly bump into him along Horse Guards Parade. His face will be rivered with tears from the effort of 26.2 miles, and the dappled shade will cover us as we embrace, two men hijacked into the story of MND in people we love.

'Where d'ya get your handle-thingy?' she says. Jo, from Walsall, is keeping pace with us and is the only person during the race who wants technical details about our wheelchair-handlebar. By the end of the conversation I'm tempted to offer to send it to her via Royal Mail. 'My daughter's nine and disabled and I want to push her in a race one day. She'd love it,' Jo says.

I can't recall the precious details of Jo's story, and by mile 23 I would feel cross with myself that so many of the names and stories of people I meet during the race have gone, such is the mental meltdown one goes through in the final stages of a marathon. But Jo impresses me. Not just that she's running the Brighton Marathon today, London Marathon next week and Manchester Marathon the week after that. There was grit in her tone, a belief that one day she will indeed push her daughter around a marathon. Another star in the constellation of resilience.

The full Brighton Marathon course replicates some of the half-marathon route, and as we continue through the city centre past St Peter's Church I'm relieved we did the half marathon as a practice. It's good to have some familiarity. I know the hill is coming and I know it will be 2 miles long. Marine Parade was an early part of the half-marathon course and I managed to get to the top without walking, so I have a precedent to follow. Two miles of ascent. According to Charlie Spedding, the tough hills are the best, and you should bound up them with an exaggerated lift of the knees and a good long push from the ankles. Well, I'm not bounding up, but the view out to sea is wonderful. The drizzle has stopped and, looking at the sky, there is brighter weather to come. Sometime during the incline my uncle receives the first of many requests for a lift, which earns us a nickname amongst the runners of 'Taxi'. We are in our rhythm. The winter and spring training is paying off. The miles seem close together, like a concertina before it fills with air. Up ahead we see a runner dressed as Noddy, with a home-made car wrapped around him.

'We must beat Noddy!' my uncle calls out. I imagine the shame of being beaten by Noddy.

We turn at the 10-mile marker and head back towards the city centre.

'That's cheating, mate!' a runner says to me. I think he's joking at first, but his face suggests otherwise. I look at my watch. It's exactly 100 minutes of running and pushing my uncle and we've just been accused of cheating. I assume it's because we've begun the descent back down the other side of Marine Parade and our pace is picking up. This is not surprising given I am struggling to stay in control. No brakes or indicators for the driver. Not even the air horn my uncle used in the half marathon to announce our arrival. That gave up the ghost before the finish in its first outing. I point out to the gentleman as he runs and tuts alongside us, that I did also do the uphills with the wheelchair. Then I do what any self-respecting runner would do. I turn on the pace and charge towards Brighton Marina, leaving him behind to eat up our NHS-tyre marks.

The city centre looms, the crowd thickens. We approach the halfway point, passing Brighton's Palace Pier. We are about to do our quickest mile of the day, at 8 minutes 38 seconds. Our injection of pace is due to a downhill mile, and the adrenalin that comes from being accused of cheating. Several times I fancy jumping on the back of the wheelchair for a ride but my first two attempts cause me to pull a wheelie. It isn't a good move. Metrically speaking, we've come 13.1 miles, but there's been a significant mental journey since our 'warm-up' half marathon here just 8 weeks ago.

'Every run has its own heartbeat,' says philosopher Mark Rowlands. I like that. No two runs are the same. The run, the person, the environment are always changing. Today's race is so different to the half marathon. The crowds are several people deep and I feel like I've had one too many bottles of raspberry energy drink. We are whooshing along, up Grand Avenue then left onto Church Road, when suddenly a television cameraman appears in front of us. I realise he's running backwards away from us. A microphone is thrust under my chin and a lady I recognise from *Women's Running* magazine, Phoebe Thomas, starts interviewing me about what's going on. I could ask her the same thing.

It becomes clear this is for Channel Four, who are doing a highlights show of the marathon, but I didn't expect us to push our way in. I tell our story as best as I can, on the move, after 14 miles, whilst trying not to do cheesy smiles at the camera and to hold in my raspberry burps. My uncle takes over the commentary. The cameraman asks us to slow down and for us to get some high-fives from the crowd – just for the camera – at precisely the moment we meet the glummest bunch of race-side dwellers we have ever seen.

Normal race protocol is that if kids raise their hands for a high-five, and you're running near the side of the road, you reciprocate. You don't initiate. Initiating high-fives went out in the days of Pheidippides (the Ancient Greek who ran from Marathon to Athens to deliver news of military victory). But now we are being filmed and this moment may be on national television next weekend. I take one hand off the wheelchair and lift it for a high-five, an attempt at audience-participation, but I swerve into the crowd and lose control, causing a grandma to leap back, a hugging couple to break apart, and a chap from B&Q to spill his tea down his front on his morning break. We fail to get a single high-five from them and the following week I find we've been edited out of the Channel Four marathon-highlights show.

We keep up the pace. People call our names. I catch a glimpse of my cousin Paul and his wife Vicky just as we pass them, waving and shouting from amid the crowd like people hailing a taxi. The next 4 miles are a loop through the residential area of Aldrington; 2 miles up to Boundary Road, then 2 miles back. A chance to spot what kind of condition those ahead of you are in, then those following you. Noddy still has a good lead on us. It's along this stretch we notice the ambulances. Several of them. There's something about their speed up the road that tells us this isn't for a guy with a dodgy ankle. There's an urgency in the air, enough for my uncle and I to both comment and express our worry.

We find out later it is tragic news. Sam Harper Brighouse, a 23-year-old man running to raise money for AIDS orphans, collapsed at the 16-mile point. At first it was thought he had experienced cardiac problems, but the post-mortem revealed it was ischemic bowel disease. About half of the runners in a marathon will get some kind of stomach trouble at some point (e.g. too many sugary products can cause problems), but this disease causes massive blood flow away from the bowel and can prove fatal. Sam possibly thought his stomach cramps were to do with the running. I've no idea if he'd experienced anything like this before or knew about it. There's nothing else the race organisers could have done. Brighton Marathon is as well organised as any I've known. The paradox is that there is a wealth of excellent advice available to runners of all levels, on nutrition, injury, kit, pacing, safety. But there will always be a minority who are underprepared, and an even smaller minority like Sam, who are just tragically unlucky. It is such a sad event, and one that understandably dominates the radio interviews I do the following day. Marathons and endurance exercise do carry risks.

'Do you think all marathon runners should see a doctor first, given the risks?' one radio host asked me.

Yes, I do. But a basic check of your blood pressure and heartbeat by a doctor with just 7 minutes allocated on their conveyer belt of appointments wouldn't eliminate many – if any – of the fatalities that happen each year. There have been more high-profile marathon deaths in recent years, mainly because there are so many more races, and more participants. It's statistically inevitable. In the marathons I've completed, I've run with a total of 160,000 people, and there have been three fatalities. One was due to hyponatremia (overhydration), one was asthma-related and the other was Sam's death.

The gurus of running say 'twenty miles is halfway'. When my uncle first told me that years ago, I thought it was rhetoric. Then I ran my first marathon and discovered its truth. We have left the vibrant noise of Brighton city centre behind and, as we head out west with the swelling sea on our left, we enter some lonely miles.

You'd never know there are hundreds of runners around us, both running out towards Shoreham power station, and a contraflow of runners heading back in. It is TOO quiet. All I hear is the pattering and muttering, as if runners feet and mouths are running out of batteries. Spectators are reduced to the occasional individual looking like a prison guard, watching us carry our suffering. There is another incline and a continuous sequence of speed bumps, which, I muse, must be designed for large armoured vehicles. At nearly 21 miles these are not fun to have to run over, less fun if you're pushing a wheelchair, and even worse if you're in the wheelchair. For my uncle, it's a different kind of endurance to what he is used to.

'Did you have a mantra to keep you going?' my wife asks me on our way home that night. I gaze out on the South Downs, the sun taking its resting place between the peaks as

I reflect on how things had turned out. Novelist Murakami says you can't survive a marathon without a mantra. I believe it can help provide focus when the brain is peering over the metaphorical cliff edge.

I had nothing rehearsed beforehand, but I did come up with a set of words that kept my mind and body together in the final 6 miles. 'Lean forward, look up, light feet.' I stick to factual instructions rather than emotional ones late on in a race, as they use up less energy. There is a physicality about our mental state. The body and mind are always in dialogue. But the dominant thought I have, after 10 months of preparation, over 500 training miles, the conversations with Hi-Viz Steve, Esther and The Man in the Red Jacket, the wheelchair training with Dennis, MicknPhil, Toby, Great Grandma and my sister, plus several parkruns in snow, is simply: 'THIS IS IT!'

We mount each speed bump and jolt back onto the road. They seem to go on forever, up and up, like a roller-coaster ride from the Stone Age. We turn the corner round the power station, past cheering race marshals, and finally we can see the sea again, raging towards us, frothing at the mouth. There are still 5 miles to go, but we know it's along the seafront and it's a psychological boost that we are now facing in the right direction. We get within reach of Noddy. I grit my teeth and surge forward, hoping to not be pulled back by PC Plod or Big Ears.

At mile 23 the crowd begins to swell, numerically and vocally. There are more shouts of our names. I realise this is it! My feet on the puddled road, my hands clenching the wheelchair. I hear the sound of my breath, rasping and keen; and the sea, clawing at the pebbles, sucking them back into itself. This is our moment, our chance. This is what we came here for. I grip my uncle's shoulder and say it as loudly as I can, above the chanting sea and the cheering crowds, 'This is it, Uncle Andrew. THIS IS IT!'

The sun is out like a gleaming silver button, spotlighting us. Not focused on the past; not seeking out the future. The sun pinpoints us in this moment. Here and Now. Free of the label of MND, our mouths full of joy and sea air. Not invisible, not forgotten, but in the race.

Then some lunatic starts yelling and waving. No, there are two, three of them. I panic that we are being pulled over or disqualified for… for… what exactly I'm not sure, but Uncle Andrew tells me he knows them. His friends, Neil and Val, are prancing like happy horses, madly swinging their hands and hats in the air with the most enormous smiles. We wave back. Their exuberance is remarkable, given they are in their seventies and not so many months ago they were attacked by cows whilst walking through a field, ending up in hospital. Just ahead of them is my uncle's son-in-law, Simon, carrying one of his children. He is not prancing like a horse, which is a relief as Simon has the London Marathon to do next week. These moments are part of the crescendo towards the finish line.

My back aches, my shoulders are tight. I have been occasionally swinging my arms round like windmills, to keep the blood flowing and avoid cramp, checking over my shoulder beforehand to avoid violence. Swinging both arms at the same time wasn't helpful for keeping on course.

'This is it, Chris. Head up, keep your chin up. Back straight, don't slouch. This is it.' I'm talking to myself, but then I hear the words replayed back to me on a loop. Uncle Andrew is repeating my pep talk. It's a team effort. I can't get through these miles without him. We reach mile 24 and the enthusiasm of the crowd is like a machine gun, encouragement being shot at us repeatedly, with so little time to say 'thank you'.

'Go guys! Whoaaaa! Go Chris and Andy!' The crowd clap, they scream, they bang the metal fencing. They are with us and for us, their desire breathing life into us.

Their noise brings me to tears. I have to put on my sunglasses for a while to stay composed. We ramp up the pace again and manage to avoid the bollards on the seafront where, in the half marathon, we had enacted a sort of reverse parking manoeuvre to get through them. Now it's just a flat coastal path all the way in.

We enter the final mile. I raise my uncle's right arm and hold it up.

'THIS IS IT!' I scream. The race marshals look puzzled, as if I am insinuating they don't know what an arm looks like. The crowd are going ballistic. I look from side to side, absorbing the ranks of unfamiliar smiling faces and the name-calling – our names – loving it and thinking 'YEEEAAAHHH!' I imagine Mick jumping up from his sofa and acting it out. The volume is phenomenal, like a radio on too loud, as we see family members and friends woven through the crowd, a mosaic of the known and the unknown cheering us on. People are loving the fact we are racing along at top speed. It's symbiotic. They scream, we speed up; we speed up and they scream louder. Palms smack the railings, whistles cut the air, so many whistles, like desperate policemen in chaotic city traffic. We overtake dozens of weary bodies in that closing mile but there's no time for pity; these other runners will have their own stories. This really is it. Today motor neurone disease is not in charge. This is a Magnificent New Day. This is us putting two fingers up at the illness. This is us, two ordinary men who love running, transforming tragedy, with the faithful weight of family urging us on, the noise of a city calling us in, and the sight of the finish line opening her arms to welcome us home. This. Is. It.

We pass the tiered seating loaded with cheering mouths and waving arms and cross the finish line, under the huge erected gantry and digital clock. We finish in 4 hours 21 minutes, ranking in the top 5,000 of those who finish. But we are more than Runners With Numbers. My uncle slowly lifts his left arm, and with all his intent pushes himself up from the wheelchair. He falls forward into me and grips me. We hug. The glorious coastal sunshine reflects off the sea of silver foil blankets wrapped around the shoulders of the finished marathoners around us.

We are enveloped in light.

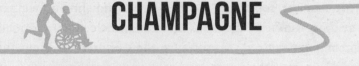

CHAMPAGNE

He who doesn't risk never gets to drink champagne.

Russian proverb

As he lifts his glass, sunlight catches the bubbles surging to the surface for breath. Uncle Andrew sits, champagne in hand, raising a toast to our marathon finish.

His three children, Sarah, Jo and Paul, stand before him, their glasses fizzing with life. Sandra is at his side. She doesn't sit down because the roast is in the oven. Their six grandchildren all play on the carpet, squirming and giggling.

My dad sits next to him, trying to make sure he doesn't knock his champagne over. Although Elizabeth can't join us, as she's back at home with a bad knee, she's been a part of this journey too. My own family is also woven into this Giant Lounge Family Tableau.

It's like the scene of the last supper, but with roast chicken to come. And nobody has a beard or sandals. A kind of Ordinary Magic has caused this coming together.

What was it Albert Einstein said about family? 'Rejoice with your family in the beautiful land of life.' I'm sure this is written somewhere near the back of my black book, but the book remains lost. It's ironic that my lists of coping strategies, words of inspiration and doodles of fish and dodgy wheels have been lost, as if testing me, causing me to rely on what lives inside me, not the ink on the pages of a book.

This 'one last marathon' has helped a family find a little bit of healing itself. It's given us something to celebrate, aided by champagne. Every family has gaps, including ours, but maybe they're getting smaller. Perhaps the healing waters of Brighton are having an effect after all.

In the midst of life's difficulties there can still be joy. Joy is not something you can bottle and stick in your understairs cupboard for the future. You can't freeze it, frame it or hang it on the wall. You can't rehearse joy. By its nature joy is always a surprise, a gift for the present moment you are in. Joy is like the champagne cork; once it's out, it's out. It arrives and sparkles in unique moments, like this.

There are clinks of glasses and coughs. Then it goes quiet.

'What was your highlight?' my dad asks. Uncle Andrew speaks first.

'Finishing has got to be a highlight, and beating Noddy,' he says. He has our attention. 'And being able to give Chris a hug at the end in the sunshine. I must say, though, it's the first race in which I've been asked to hold cold salted potatoes.'

More champagne is poured. 'What about sitting in the wheelchair for all that time?' Sarah asks.

'Sitting in the wheelchair for nearly five hours was no problem. No sore bottom thankfully.' He looks up and smiles. Nobody asks for evidence to back up the claim. Some things can be taken on trust. 'My neck got stiff but that is fairly common now, not because of sitting in the wheelchair. I had to trust Chris to see the upcoming potholes and bollards. I didn't want to keep on saying "mind this, mind that". Fortunately Chris did see them...' He pauses. 'Um... except one... but I won't mention that.' Then he hands me a wrapped box. It is the gift of a glass tankard on which the words 'Brighton Marathon. A Great Push!' are inscribed. When I get home I test it out. It works fine with cider or beer; this tankard isn't fussy.

The grandchildren get restless, as we relive the ending of the race.

'The atmosphere along the final stretch was incredible,' he says. He looks like he is back in the moment. 'It was so noticeable that when people saw us they gave an extra cheer and the volume went up. That brought a tear to my eye. I think because Chris was steaming along at such a rate of knots, that impressed the crowd and increased the noise level.' I admit I got carried away and stopped looking for potholes, bollards and other runners' ankles.

'This journey has been really hard, to be honest with you,' my uncle says. 'It's been emotional, but it's also had times of being good fun and really rewarding.' Those words he uttered after his disastrous 1996 London Marathon are relevant once again. 'You know, I can't go out on a low note.'

In the days after the race, friends, family and strangers tell us they have entered their first races. They're training for 5-km and 10-km races, half and full marathons. They're getting their kit on and going out the door more often, which is preferable to getting their kit off and going out the door more often. Several weeks after our Brighton Marathon, my neighbour, Murray, proudly completes his first run, of less than a mile to the village traffic lights and back. All 114 kilograms (18 stone) of him. Nine months later he completes the London Marathon for the first time in his life.

We want our story to shed light on life with MND, and stir a passion for running. I think we've made a start. Perhaps the journey has not ended. Endings can be as unpredictable as beginnings, as events across the Atlantic showed the day immediately after the race.

BOSTON SPEAKS

It's so much darker when a light goes out than
it would have been if it had never shone.

John Steinbeck

Scaffolding twists and falls. Windows spew out their glass, like a deafening sneeze. Bodies collapse in unison amid sounds of confusion. Hanging shredded and forlorn are the blue flags of the Boston Athletics Association.

***

It is an attack unprecedented in sporting history, blood marking the street in a signature of terrorism. Two pressure-cooker bombs, constructed out of old oven parts by young Russian brothers with a grudge against their immigrant home of North America. Home-made bombs filled with nails and ball bearings, and placed in rucksacks near the finish line of the most historic marathon in the world. Two bombs,

THE REASON I RUN

a hundred metres apart, detonated within 30 seconds of each other.

Two brothers, two bombs, too much.

The impact of those two bombs at the Boston Marathon finish line on Boylston Street, the day after the Brighton Marathon, ripple across the Atlantic and connect our story irrevocably to theirs.

As news of the attack unfolds, I am in my lounge halfway through writing up events from our race, my legs aching, toes blistered, hands black from the gloves. My head is still full of tigers, green telephones and the tragedy which had occurred in the Brighton race. I sit confused, watching BBC Breaking News, my mouth open. Images are on repeat from Boylston Street: emergency-services personnel in hi-viz gear assist wounded runners and distressed spectators. Different news reporters provide the same sound bites.

Martin Richard had wanted to see his dad finish the race so he climbed onto the metal railing on Boylston Street to get a better view. He became the youngest victim of the bombing, just 8 years old. A father and son torn apart at the finish line. In the explosion Martin's 6-year-old sister, Jane, lost a leg and was unconscious for 2 weeks. His mum, Denise, lost vision in one eye and required head surgery. His marathon-running dad, Bill, lost part of his hearing from shrapnel and, although this will return in time, he lost much on that one day. Only Martin's big brother, Henry, escaped without physical injury, but his family was devastated. How does a family respond after such loss?

Given the explosions and mayhem, not everyone finished the Boston Marathon that day. That's not unusual for a marathon with the ever-present enemies of fatigue, dehydration and injury, but on this tragic day, with shattered glass and bags deserted in a hurry, a no-go zone was formed. Weary runners were turned back and no amount of defiance would get them through.

Two who didn't finish the race were Boston locals Dick and Rick Hoyt. Dick and Rick are a father-and-son team, with Dick pushing his son Rick in his wheelchair. They completed their first marathon in 1981 – the same year as the first London Marathon. Rick was deprived of oxygen when he was born and diagnosed as a spastic quadriplegic with cerebral palsy.

'People said to us, "Forget him. Put him away. He's just a vegetable," but he's in his fifties now and we still haven't worked out what vegetable he is,' says Dick.

When he was fifteen, Rick told his dad, speaking with the help of a computer, that he wanted to participate in a 5-mile benefit run for a friend who had been paralysed in an accident. His dad agreed to push Rick in his wheelchair. They came in next to last.

That night, Rick told his dad, 'When we're running, it feels like I'm not handicapped.' So they kept going. They didn't stop, not even at marathons. They have completed duathlons (cycling and running) and triathlons (swimming, cycling, running), of which six have been Ironman competitions. In a triathlon, for the swimming stage Dick will pull his son in a boat with a bungee cord attached from the front of the boat to his waist. For the biking phase, Rick will ride in a special two-seater bicycle with his dad, and in the running stage Dick will push Rick in his custom-made running chair. How far is the running stage in an Ironman? A full marathon. Seeing them in action is a moving picture of resilience in every sense of that phrase.

Rick was once asked, if he could give his father one thing, what would it be?

'The thing I'd most like is for my dad to sit in the chair and I would push him for once,' he said.

On crossing a thousand finish lines together, Dick purchased a restaurant and called it 'The Finishing Line'. Speaking to *The New York Times*, Rick said, 'When my dad and I are out there on a run, a special bond forms between us and it feels like there is nothing Dad and I cannot do.' I'd like to imagine my uncle and I as an English incarnation of Dick and Rick Hoyt, but with 999 less finish lines. They are Champions League; as a wheelchair-pusher, I am Conference League.

Boston remains special for Rick and Dick, the place of their first marathon and one they have completed 30 times. They are unstoppable. Unstoppable, that is, until a home-made bomb goes off when they're at mile 23 and have to be turned back.

Dick and Rick Hoyt decided they weren't done. Tragedy was not going to stop them. The following day, their heads still full of the news and Dick's legs still full of lactate acid, they headed out on to the marathon route. Again. All of it. The fatigue from 23 miles of running and pushing the previous day wasn't enough to squash their defiance.

'People came out of their homes and cheered us on; it was amazing,' said Dick. They crossed the finish line to complete another Boston Marathon. Father and son, proud at the finish line.

Watching events in Boston, it's clear there's no line between us and them. While the tragedy was over 3,000 miles away, to runners it feels personal. It is an attack on the running community, on OUR values, OUR way of celebrating life in sweat-wicking gear. By the time the morning papers arrive at the newsagents, it is evident that terrorism was the cause. Or, more specifically, two brothers, one in a white cap, the other in a black cap. Two brothers attempting to drain the light out of a city, the colour out of a nation, the courage out of a community of people who run for their lives. They tried to take our breath away, but they picked the wrong people. If tragedy creates connections, running only makes them stronger.

Resilience doesn't mean rising effortlessly above difficulties, like a helium balloon. It pulses at the heart of all our stories. It's a thread through all our lives, holding us together when tragedy tries to tear us apart, better than gaffer tape and plastic tags. It's true for individuals, but also for places and communities: Brighton on 12 October 1984; New York on 11 September 2001; London on 7 July 2005; Boston on 15 April 2013. Pick your place, you'll find people knitting their lives back together. Families and communities knowing they need each other.

Events in Boston remind me running is not about the numbers. I hear again those words over the loudspeaker as my son ran with me down the Shakespeare Marathon home straight, 'RUNNER WITH NO NUMBER.' When it comes down to it, it's not just about distance covered, speed accomplished, finishing time achieved or position gained. I love busting my limits, picking off fellow runners round the final bend and propelling myself like a lunatic in an attempt to take a single second off my PB. But that's not the whole story. Numbers provide rhythm, but they're not the melody. It's not just what you do, but why you do it. Not just your results, but also your reasons.

After a disturbed night, I drive to work, visuals and voices from Boston replaying in my mind. Blossom, discarded by the wind, drifts across the road in front of me. I accelerate down the A46 and over the River Arrow. I glance across at the river; it's always in motion, always alive. If you look carefully, the river, like life, is never on repeat.

As I drive to my first school visit for the day, men in suits zoom past, hurrying away, ignorant of the speed limit. I wonder what questions about the events in Boston my friend David would be asking if he was in my passenger seat today.

I enter the village and turn up the high street and drive over freshly painted speed bumps. So much easier in a car than with a wheelchair. I arrive just as registration is being completed. The bell sounds and the corridor fills with young people talking, swinging schoolbags, jostling for their place, shambling towards elsewhere.

First off I meet with a 16-year-old boy in the corner of his school cafeteria, to hear how he is coping. His dad is ill with cancer and has itchy hands from chemotherapy. My role today is listening, letting him take the conversation where he wants to. Today he talks about bicycles, because the reality of his dad's situation is too much for him. Sometimes talking about difficulties makes them feel real and the truth is you don't always feel defiant; sometimes you just want to switch off. 'Automatic' doesn't make room for chemotherapy.

Afterwards I drive to another school 8 miles away, listening to BBC Radio 5 Live in the car. They're talking about yesterday's bombing in Boston. I arrive with 10 minutes to spare and park badly on a kerb in the school car park. I flick through my session notes from last week and get ready to meet four teenage boys, one after the other, dealing with issues from anxiety to punching holes in school walls; from being on the run from a violent father to not being fussed about education (but expressed in stronger language).

'Girls ask for help, boys act for help,' says psychologist Stephen Biddulph.

I turn the radio off. A Twitter notification announces itself on my phone. It's from a stranger. The phone sits illuminated on my passenger seat. I hesitate, my work bag and notes balancing on my lap, then I reach for it.

The message is from a researcher, called Laura, at BBC Radio 5 Live, asking for my comments about the bombing in Boston. She can't have known I was listening to the show. Laura has contacted two people to speak live on air. One of them is Liz Yelling, British Olympic runner and Commonwealth Games bronze medallist. The other is me, who came second behind Christian Dinnage in the 1,500-metre race at school sports day 23 years ago.

I call Laura. I explain how things turned out with my uncle barely 48 hours ago. She thinks I have something to say, then tells me she'd like my comments live on air in precisely 7 minutes' time. I sprint from the car, in shiny black shoes with no cushioning, and burst into the school reception. I tell Donna at the front desk that I need a room urgently – but not the bathroom, and follow her instructions. I run up four flights of stairs, coat still on, to find a quiet space where I can do the radio interview. I find a room. A small square room used for storing retired computers and disused telephones. There's a soft chair in the corner. I sit down and try to get my breath back, breathing in through my nose while counting to three, trying to think about not panicking. Which means I am thinking about panicking. Then I count to six as I breathe out, like I'm blowing up a balloon. My feet are planted apart on the carpet, like tree roots going into the ground. That's precisely how I describe to boys the process they should carry out when they feel anxious or cross. How to ground themselves. Now I'm having to take my own advice. I wait my turn on national radio, hoping the phone signal will be OK, checking out the broken phones in the box at my elbow. Will the connection hold?

I am still out of breath when the familiar voice of radio host Nicky Campbell comes on.

'So, Chris from Warwickshire, are you… are you an athlete?' he says. It's a good question, behind which others queue for attention, like: Do you run? Why did you start? What matters to you about it? What's your personal-best time? Runners love hunting for numbers.

My debut on national radio begins with me breathing heavily down the phone, suggesting I may not be the athlete Nicky is looking for. I try to compose myself, sweating in my coat, and start telling Nicky my story. A story about my uncle, a doddery wheelchair, a marathon and an illness that will kill him too soon. A story not just about us as runners, but as people connected to a community which stretches across every continent. An army of people who believe the gift of Ordinary Magic is available to all.

Tragedy in Boston the day after triumph in Brighton brought many stories together. We are runners. We keep going.

MY UNCLE
AND THE TREE

There is no such thing as an ending.
Just the place where we choose to stop the story.

Frank Herbert

A week after the Brighton race, aware of the heightened sense of alarm resulting from the Boston explosions on the Monday, I go to London. It's surreal to be there as a spectator for the world's greatest race, seeing Mo Farah on his teasing debut (deliberately stopping at halfway), and more aware than ever of the elite wheelchair racers. I watch Paralympians, including double amputee Richard Whitehead springing along on his prosthetics. I love the London Marathon. Look beyond the big brands and million-pound sponsorship, and you'll find a colourful celebration of joy, movement and humanity. An enormous experience for anyone.

The race provides an exciting climax in the men's elite race as 2011 champion Emmanuel Mutai, from Kenya, looks to have it sealed with a mile and a half to go. But then Ethiopian Tsegaye Kebede, running with his elbows sticking out, finishes strongly, and wins by 30 seconds.

At the end of the race my uncle and I meet up by a tree, sunlight fracturing through the leaves. It is not any old tree where we meet. The tree is in the repatriation area for marathon finishers, near Horse Guards Parade. We are celebrating family members who have completed today's marathon: my wife, Cousin Paul, Uncle Andrew's son-in-law Simon and my good friend Sam are all meeting here, each hobbling through the crowd, Virgin-red goody bags in hand, tear-streaked cheeks and medals proudly worn. They arrive at intervals, depending on their finish time. Somewhere still out there on the course is Hi-Viz Steve and a man called Mark Maddox, attempting to be the first person living with MND to complete the London Marathon on foot. Mark told me afterwards that doctors had warned him the chances of completing it were stacked against him due to the effects of the disease on his body. But he went ahead anyway.

'I'm a positive person,' he says, 'and my mind is my biggest weapon in the fight against the illness. I see the faces of my kids and they keep me inspired and that's enough for me.' He completes it in 6 hours 40 minutes, a phenomenal achievement.

Here we are, at last, completing a full circle from 6 years earlier when my uncle and I failed to meet up after running the same marathon for the first time. Not knowing then that our next one together would be with a wheelchair smothered in gaffer tape and the reality of a life-limiting illness to contend with.

I stand next to him in his wheelchair. We get talking about our race a week ago.

'So what comes next?' he asks. It's the question on both our minds, but which neither has spoken until now.

We stand shaded from the sun, in a kind of daylight darkness. An in-between place. So what comes next? I start to wonder what it would be like to do just one more race together...

THE MAGIC OF MOVEMENT

All that is important is this one moment in movement.
Do not let it slip away unnoticed and unused.

Martha Graham

The Brighton Marathon was supposed to be my uncle's last race. But it doesn't work out that way.

We get together for the undulating Kenilworth Half Marathon in September that year, the same race that Hi-Viz Steve and Crash Helmet Judy had completed the previous year. We start last, after giving a short interview to BBC Coventry and Warwickshire radio, then go out and wreck our personal-best time from the Brighton Half Marathon, reducing it by 6 minutes (finishing in 1 hour 54 minutes). I feel out of control on the descents.

'No brakes!' we both yell as we torpedo our way through from the back. My brother-in-law Graham runs his first half marathon on the day, overtaking us on the uphills and watching us pass like a blur on the downhills. He also finishes in well under 2 hours.

Then we take on the Brighton Half Marathon again for the second year in a row, once more encountering problems about the validity of our entry (with race manager Paul coming to the rescue again). On the only sunny day in February, we knock another minute off our PB, starting at the front again with a 30-second head start. We dash past the seafront beach huts, smashed to pieces by the previous week's storms.

'Come on, Chris, leave it on the road,' I say aloud to myself in the final mile, swerving between other weary-legged runners.

'Just as long as you don't leave me on the road,' replies my uncle, gripping the wheelchair with his left hand as we stampede towards the finish line.

Then we sign up to our second full marathon, in Worcester in May, a little over a year since our Brighton Marathon. The race is organised by Tempo Events, who had hosted the Scorpion Run earlier in the year. On a warm bank holiday weekend, with a small field of about 250 marathoners (plus about 750 doing the half marathon), we encounter what seems to be every hill Worcestershire has to offer.

We pull over at 7 miles because my uncle wants the banana from his coat pocket. Note to uncle: never store a ripe banana in a coat pocket on a hot day.

'Yeeeugh!' he says, removing his hand from the pocket to reveal a layer of yellow pulp smeared upon it. I wipe his hand clean with a tissue. Even in his forty-first marathon there is something to learn.

We unexpectedly meet Mick and Phil spectating halfway round and stop for a chat, at which point a lady in front of us falls, twisting her ankle and calling out in agony. She is slumped in the road on a sharp bend, and the country roads are still open to traffic, so we do our best to help her. Between us we finally get a marshal in a car to collect her and take her safely to the finish.

Given that most runners are doing the half marathon, the second lap is sparsely populated and as expected we find ourselves near the back. We chat to other runners, Kate and Big Rich from the 100 Marathon Club for whom running a marathon is a regular part of their weekend activity, and Sally, who is also running for the MND Association. She lost a friend to the disease just months before.

'I've got MND,' my uncle explains to her and tells her our story. 'Story-telling pace' should be an official pacing category.

Our family keep appearing en route, outside pubs, in lay-bys, by canal bridges, cheering us on. My dad with his camera, Elizabeth, Sandra and Jo with their cheering, my wife with our three high-spirited children in check. They tell spectators our story and people spontaneously give them money for the MND Association. Others go home afterwards and sign the MND Charter. Hope is infectious. Stories kick us into action more than statistics, perhaps because we find ourselves mirrored in the story, separated from the numbers.

'Chris! Chris!' someone is shouting as they sprint down a hill at mile 14, a hill we are trying to run up. It only becomes clear when she is within arm's reach that it is my sister. She joins us in her running kit and runs with us for 5 miles – a runner with no number – but she gets cheered on like the rest of us. I confess to her that I have a craving for coffee-and-walnut cake. My body is subconsciously saying it wants carbs, caffeine, minerals and sugar (cake craving is highly scientific). She leaves us at mile 19, drives 40 minutes home, makes a fantastic coffee-and-walnut cake and brings it to our family gathering later that afternoon.

At mile 22 my uncle spots a tree riddled with mistletoe.

'Don't kiss me,' he shouts over his shoulder. But I stop under the tree, not heeding his command, and kiss the back of his head, my way of saying 'thank you' for holding my tub of cold salted potatoes once again.

Then two young ladies in a Mini holler at us with a toy megaphone through their half-wound-down window. They pull to the side of the road and blast out 'Eye of the Tiger' on their stereo as we shuffle past – the perfect soundtrack for where our wheelchair-marathon racing started, back in Brighton's Preston Park, my daughter looking scared by a carbon-fibre creature. They seek us out at the finish line and tell us their story about a friend they lost to MND just a few weeks ago. It's the Iceberg Principle: we saw a Mini parking badly and heard the Rocky theme tune cranked up way too loud. But beneath the surface: Tragedy, Running, Connections. No Them and Us.

As we reach 26 miles, we turn from the canal path toward the towering Sixways rugby stadium, home of Worcester Warriors, where the inflatable finishing archway is situated. I see my kids, waiting. Caleb runs and claps alongside us; Maisie-Joy skips; Toby, with his 3-year-old legs, tries to keep up and not get in the way of my dodgy steering. I lift my uncle's arm to acknowledge the crowd and our families, trying not to lose control, pushing him one-handed around the final bend. He has lost the strength to keep his head up. It has been an exhausting race. With my uncle in front, and my children beside, we cross the line, together.

We finish the hilly race in 4 hours 59 minutes. It was never about the finish time, but the Whole Time. We expected the Worcester Marathon to be our last race.

MND is not an illness any of us want to keep quiet about. Later that day we get messages of congratulations from people in the public eye who don't want to keep quiet about it either. TV and radio host Nicky Campbell; TV presenter Nick Knowles; runner Nell McAndrew; Olympian Jo Pavey; TV and radio presenter Zoe Ball. Uncle Andrew is moved to be remembered by so many, lending their strength and lifting his spirits.

I'm convinced all the resources we need to get through whatever we face are within us, around us and available to us. When we lend our strength to others it multiplies. This doesn't eliminate struggles or despair, but it means we can find something lasting in the depths of them.

'Love attempts things beyond its strength,' wrote Thomas à Kempis. My uncle's positive mindset is exemplary, but he is still human and the reality of MND brings tricky, sad and devastating days for him and all the family. In the months to come Paul will tell me about needing to help his dad put his jacket on, lifting one heavy arm at a time, doing up the zip for him, turning the collar. What a father once did for his son, now reversed. There are days when Uncle Andrew will walk delicately into the kitchen using his walking frame and sob into his wife's arms. When the illness just feels too much, and unfair. At their home, handrails have been fixed by the front door, the stairlift is fitted, and the occupational therapist visits to monitor his needs. There is a shower seat in the bathroom, and two walking frames – one upstairs and one downstairs. The illness is no longer just present in conversation and thought, but in apparatus which get in the way, squeak and leave marks on the carpet. The MND Association have helped pay for some of this equipment.

'The main change is a weakening of my legs. I can no longer walk without my frame. I'm unable to walk from the house to the car without help,' he tells me. From the house to the car is his new marathon distance.

'I've also developed a cough, which I think is due to weakening throat muscles,' he says, 'and I've been wearing my neck brace the last few days.' This means a permanent change.

I email him with some questions about a marathon he once competed in, and he replies to telephone him instead. 'I can just about type two lines for an email,' he says to me, 'but after that I struggle to keep my hands on the keyboard. My fingers cramp up.'

Life continues, and changes, as the illness quietly invades more territory of his body. He knows, from running 39 marathons or longer, plus completing two in his wheelchair, that you can only deal with the mile you're in. Each one a little tougher than the last.

I try to figure out where our story goes next. Do we lead it or does it lead us?

On our wedding anniversary in September, my wife and I take on the Cheltenham Half Marathon together, the town where I got my first ever running trainers and learned how to pronounce the brand names. It is my seventeenth attempt at trying to conquer 1 hour 30 minutes. It is perfect running weather, through the striking colours of late summer and cool air. But I am worried I've overdone my preparation, as only last weekend I ran 41 miles in less than 24 hours at the inaugural Spitfire Scramble, London's first off-road 24-hour race. I'd run as a pair with Hannah, taking it in turns to run loops of 5.8 miles around Hornchurch Country Park in east London. It was brilliant fun, but not the recommended approach a week before a race where you're hungry for a PB.

Just under 3,000 people stand on the start line in Cheltenham. I risk being near the front. Alas, I don't have a 30-second head start. Halfway round I am just 40 seconds up on my target time. I spring up the hill at mile 8 at 6-minutes-51-seconds-per-mile pace, exactly the pace I need to be running. I stick with it on the lonely lap around the racecourse at mile 10, then lose 20 seconds with the undulations. A PB is within reach, I keep telling myself. Then with a mile to go, as the sun comes out strongly, I can feel my legs tightening up. Mentally, I am wobbling. A short man in a Cambridge Triathlon Club top overtakes me; his leg turnover is impressive. Cambridge: in my mind I hear the cello of Messiaens, I see the black-and-white floor of Pembroke College, I think of David's Lotus Elise. Speed. Speed! SPEED IS WHAT I NEED!

'You've got great cadence,' I say to the gentleman in the Cambridge top as he speeds past. I didn't mean it as a chat-up line, but he turns round and beckons me to run with him. He becomes the horse, I am the cart. Up an ascent at mile 12 we run together, him checking on me over his shoulder, then past the final water station. I have no time to collect water. We carve our way through the grounds of Pittville Pump Rooms with half a mile to go. As much as I have enjoyed the views of the Cotswold hills and blue sky in the first half of the race, I had run with constant attention to my watch. My pace. My numbers. My chance. I turn the final corner before a downhill finish along a tree-lined avenue. With a tired brain I do the sums, like Tom the Blacksmith with his giant calculator: 12.84 miles are done, just 0.26 to go. I see the digital clock ahead.

I grit my teeth for another bad finish-line photo, and sprint for my life. High knees. Pumping arms. The crowd deafening my pain. I finish 121st out of 2,944 finishers but the numbers that matter to me are on my watch: 1 hour 29 minutes 39 seconds. I have finally cracked it.

While other runners tamely walk through the finishing funnel of metal railings, muttering and glancing at their watch, I jump up and down screaming delight.

'Yes! YEEEEESS!' Like I am the Lottery winner. The Big Finger is pointing at ME! My laughter shakes the trees. The Numbers are a drug and I am falling under their spell.

Cambridge Man waits for me. 'Thank you,' I say, 'I was done for, but you got me through that last mile.'

We talk for several minutes as we stretch our legs by the railings. He is my new hero, so I copy his routine.

'I'm Chris, by the way,' I say. We shake hands, another strong grip.

'Good to meet you. I'm Andrew,' he says. I laugh. Once again, an Andrew crosses the line immediately before me. Then my wife comes through with a race PB of 1 hour 39 minutes, taking 3 minutes off her previous PB, and therefore technically closing the gap on Mo Farah, who wins the Great North Run on the same day in 1 hour, 0 minutes, 1 second.

A week after our race is an event to celebrate 10 years of the mentoring work of Lifespace Trust, the project my friend David thought would fail. A decade of helping reduce the distress of over a thousand individual young people, and building their resilience. I decide to go public on an idea I've been carrying for a while, and announce my attempt to run ten marathons in 10 days, to raise £10,000 for the charity. The numerical symmetry is satisfying, although I don't think my legs will be as happy. Someone tells me they think it's a ridiculous idea. Someone else predicts I'll fail after number four and 'end up all disappointed with myself'. They might be right, but I'm a runner. Resistance makes me stronger. Hi-Viz Steve is going to run with me on day 10, as will friends from Lifespace and some of my family. I might fail, but that has to be a possibility for it to mean something. Uncle Andrew plans to be there to cheer me on, no doubt wishing he'd brought his electric socks with him. As I finish writing, I am in training, my wife teaching me how to do proper core-stability exercises. So my personal running performance still has some big goals to go for, but the journey with Uncle Andrew isn't over. A few weeks after the Worcester Marathon I hear from Summersdale, who say they love the story and want to go ahead and publish. I text my uncle with the exciting news. His reply? 'Fantastic. Any news on Oxford?' He definitely has his sights on another race.

I had started investigating the Oxford Half Marathon, as it is a mostly flat single-lap course. It passes the Mini plant facility in Cowley, then continues to the Iffley Road athletics track, where Sir Roger Bannister ran the first ever sub-4-minute mile in May 1954.

To celebrate the sixtieth anniversary of Bannister's famous 3:59.4 mile, the half-marathon race will include a single lap of the track so runners will get 'the unique opportunity to run in Bannister's footsteps', say the organisers. The course takes in the city's historical university grounds and the 'dreaming spires' which dominate the skyline, like fingers pointing to higher places. Oxford is a place which makes you lift your head. The race skirts Christ Church Meadow, before crossing Folly Bridge onto the scenic (but slightly potholed) Thames

Path. The finish line is in the Kassam Stadium, home of Oxford United Football Club.

I confess I have a soft spot for Oxford. It sings with history, its road names are full of majesty: King Edward St, Queen St, St Aldate's. As a runner from Shakespeare's Stratford, I will relish racing along streets where C. S. Lewis and J. R. R. Tolkien have walked. Did they ever watch Bannister run? Who knows? In my mind, Oxford marries running and story-telling. A fitting finale to our journey, perhaps.

I email Uncle Andrew with details and photographs of the terrain and obstacles to negotiate, especially the bumpy Thames Path.

'I'm sure we can manage it. Overcoming obstacles is what this is all about,' he says. Whereas a year before he could have clambered out of the wheelchair and walked a quarter of a mile, now he can't. The wheelchair is a fixture.

And so it comes to be on a cold October day that we have a racing quartet, as two of his children, Sarah and Paul, agree to run with us. The traffic into Oxford is a nightmare, causing a delay to the start of the race. I leave my own family stuck in the traffic and run a mile and a half down the central reservation to get to the bus collection point. I arrive out of breath to find a queue of over 500 people for the buses. We, the running quartet, finally locate each other at the start, but the race is already underway. We have missed Sir Roger Bannister starting it and we cross the line with three spectators watching. We can see a couple of runners about 200 metres ahead. It is something of an anticlimax. But we slowly close the gap, stopping briefly at mile 3 to put a neck support on Uncle Andrew, as he is finding it hard to keep his head up. Sarah pushes her dad around the lap of the Iffley

Road track and Paul pushes for at least half the race, pressing on ahead of Sarah and myself. Our families are noisy at the roadside and again at the end, where we finish in an almost empty Kassam Stadium. I hold my uncle's arm aloft, our signature finish on the home straight, and we finish in 2 hours 32 minutes. We are immediately accosted by a local reporter for the *Oxford Mail*. It has been a rather incognito race for us, but the chance to tell the story is a welcome lift. Our day ends with nearly all the family (plus 40 other runners) waiting at the designated bus stop for a lift back to the Mini plant nearly 2 miles away where our cars are parked. The bus never arrives (an apology from the race organisers does eventually). So a day that began with a 15-minute run to the start line finishes with a half-hour walk back, with six tired children in tow. Hardly the fitting finale I'd hoped for.

But Paul had finally got the chance to race with his dad.

In fact, it leads to a wonderful, unexpected next step. A few weeks after the chaos of the Oxford race, Paul secures two places in the next Brighton Marathon. One for him, one for his dad in his rickety but race-wise wheelchair.

'I know this will be our final chance,' Paul says.

I ask my uncle for his thoughts. 'I wasn't expecting another marathon after the epic in Worcester,' he says, 'but when Paul asked, having taken me out for a run and push on Boxing Day, I knew I couldn't let him down.'

Finally, father and son, a racing duo.

* * *

What is the message my uncle has been living out? He's taught me to live like I'm running at my best. With my head up, leaning into the day I'm given. To cherish the body I'm resident in and encourage others along the way. To remember that some miles are for enjoying, while others are for enduring, but that we should live them all until the finish, always searching for our personal best.

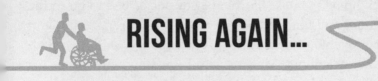

RISING AGAIN...

I collapse to the ground. A lady at my side gasps. A child points his finger at me. I look up and see the digital clock ticking... ticking... The finish line of the Beachy Head Marathon is within sight, at the bottom of a steep 60-metre hill. Beyond that are more Sussex cliffs with October sunshine spilling its gold upon them, the horizon, and then who knows what? My uncle Andrew had inspired me to attempt this race.

'It's one of the toughest in England,' he'd told me earlier in the year. It used to be his favourite race when he could still run. Right now, it looks as if I won't quite make it.

* * *

Only a few weeks before I'd been in Warwick Hospital. 'We need to work out what's going on with your heart. We think you may have had a mild heart attack,' the doctor had said.

What had led to me being rushed into hospital? The day before I'd run 22 miles in training in 3 hours, feeling like I had superhero powers. I had run my heart out, as I knew I had a minor operation coming up, involving local anaesthetic and a surgeon who resembled the serial murderer Dr Harold Shipman. This was concerning, as that same surgeon now held a scalpel and a blowtorch. As I lay on a trolley in a whitewashed room, underwear around my ankles, I reminded myself I didn't want to create any more children.

Back home the next morning I got out of bed to go to the bathroom and fainted. On the toilet. I was trapped upright, preventing blood getting to my brain. My kids rushed to fetch my neighbour, Murray, who helped my wife lift me off the toilet, but I was in and out of consciousness for half an hour. Murmuring nonsense. Head flopping. Body in spasm. Paramedics came, shaved my chest, attached pads with wires, and got a dodgy heart-reading printout to analyse. Welcome Back To Warwick Hospital.

It had, unsurprisingly, made me question whether I should do the off-road marathon on the Sussex coast several weeks later. After the scans and monitoring were done, and I was certain the passing out was due to a combination of anaesthetic from the previous day's op, and me being bradycardic (low heart rate) in the first place, I decided to go ahead. I don't advise this, but it's what I did. I had a good stack of training miles in the tank and promised my wife I'd be sensible and check my pulse at every checkpoint.

I took it steady and, true to my word, checked my pulse regularly, whilst eating pastries and chocolate. I could have happily decamped at some of those checkpoints. Uncle Andrew, Auntie Sandra and Cousin Jo came and cheered me on along the route at Birling Gap, and again in the closing 2 miles along the cliff top after I'd suffered the Seven Sisters hills, running (not walking) them all.

Then I see the inflatable finish line, beyond the final 60-metre descent. So with tired legs from nearly 4.5 hours of trail running, I collapse to the ground. But everything is OK. This is self-inflicted drama, a choice made with my heart full of joy. As spectators gasp, I take a leaf out of my son's book and re-enact his elaborate signature finish, doing a triple roly-poly down the hill. Onlookers are relieved − not that they know about my heart reading or the purple swelling in my shorts − before breaking out into applause as I roll and tumble over the turf, over and over. I rise again and stagger the final steps across the finish line, with muddy stripes on the back of my fluorescent orange top, like tiger marks. Good job my daughter isn't here. I finish in 4 hours 22 minutes, 1 minute longer than the Brighton Marathon took with my uncle earlier in the year.

Having crossed the line in one piece, I queue for a post-race hot chocolate and look around. You can smell the coming storm in the air.

I walk through the patchwork of runners spread out on the grass, basking in the warmth, the weight of medals pressing in on their chests. I lean on a railing and look across at the cliffs, daunting and steadfast, land formed by the sea and moulded by the elements.

'It helps... to step back and take a long view,' wrote Archbishop Oscar Romero. He reminds us we shouldn't expect to be able to do everything. We are not designed to. We can draw on strength from beyond ourselves, for none of us are superhuman. Our contribution may be a fraction of what is required, but it is still essential. 'This enables us to do something, and do it well,' he said.

I stand, watching the waves below rushing in, then pulling themselves back, not sure whether they are arriving or departing. Each wave rises, peaks and breaks, part of a greater ocean. I listen to my breathing. Rising, falling, rising again, like miniature resurrections.

'You don't win a battle because of how it turns out. You win by the way you face it,' said Rosie Swale Pope, my Queen of Ordinary Magic. What did I write in her black book, that day I met her with her trailer outside the garage? From what I remember, it was that life contains loss, but there is always a reason to keep going. To be brave and contemplate that there can still be good things ahead, tucked away out of sight in the future. Sometimes you have to go searching for them. Sometimes they find you. My uncle will win his battle, not because his prognosis will change, but because of how he is facing the illness. Living each mile to the full. Bringing a family together when tragedy tried to tear it apart.

I grip the rail and inhale the coastal air. I stare at where the sky and sea touch.

'D'you see it? D'you see it now?' Skip would say if he were here, his long arm outstretched, pointing toward the horizon. I try and figure out how far away it is, but that's not where my attention needs to be. Life is not there, out of reach. It's here, at hand. It's Now.

ACKNOWLEDGEMENTS

Stories are born and thrive in the community and so many people have contributed to ours.

Thank you Uncle Andrew for your 100-per-cent dedication at every twist and turn of this journey. What a privilege to have raced with you, and to have got to know you more. Thank you for your example of resilience and service and for all the coaching advice too. Thank you Auntie Sandra for your hospitality and tireless support, and Sarah, Paul and Jo for trusting me with your dad, in snow, rain and heatwaves. Thank you Jo for all the photos.

Thank you Hannah who knows what this has meant to me and required behind the scenes. Without your incredible support I wouldn't have even started. Thank you for backing me, and inspiring me, and for your sacrifices along the way, especially when I was frequently writing through the night. And running through the night. You are amazing. To Caleb, Maisie-Joy and Toby, I love watching you run, such smiles and determination. You all rock! Be curious about all the good things you can make happen.

To Helen, Graham, Jack and Ollie, thank you for cake, colourful banners, amazing support and the chances to run together. To Dad and Elizabeth, thank you for your constancy and enthusiasm. You all gave us strength when none was left. We couldn't have asked for more faithful support.

To all those mentioned in the story who helped me train, and learn some kind of control over a wheelchair at speed. Thank you for your patience, insights and encouragement. To Mick and Phil Curry, Steve Atherton, Sue and Dennis, Great

Grandma Esther Osborne (I hope your nerves have settled now). To Steve Clifford for the surprise cheque to buy my first pair of proper running shoes. To Jess Thomas and Tom the Blacksmith for the wheelchair handlebar contraption. It's had a lot of use and you were both patient and generous. Thank you Joanna Robinson for the sports massages and introduction to new forms of pain, a.k.a. stretching.

I've spoken to (emailed, tweeted, skyped, had coffee with, etc.) many people who know the daily reality of MND in their lives, homes and families far better than I do. Thank you for helping me learn more and inspiring me with your resilience, honesty and humour. You are: Eric and Davina Rivers, Liam Dwyer, Louise Oswald, Sarah Ezekiel, Mark Maddox, Esther Roberts. Thank you to The Revd. Michael Wenham and Monarch Books for permission to draw on your personal experience of MND. And to Lindy Jones, I wish you could have read this story before you left us. Also in memory of Nikki Woodman and Ludo Garcia, our thoughts are with your families MND took you from.

To Rosie Swale Pope, it was a joy to cross paths with you, and Rory Coleman for all the advice when I took on my first ultra. To Murray next door. You've got a sub-5-hour marathon in there somewhere. To the many runners who shared the miles with us, especially in Brighton, and made us laugh so much. It's true, Brighton rocks. Thank you also to Horsham Joggers for all the ways you've enriched my uncle's running life, and to Horsham Lions too.

To all my friends and the team at Lifespace Trust, especially Mike for listening so much. To all the young men I've had the privilege to mentor, who through their own stories have enriched my idea and experience of resilience.

Thank you Danny Coyle for helping me believe this story was worth telling, and the opportunity through *Men's Running* magazine to do so. To the incredible team at Summersdale for your enthusiasm from the start and spot-on advice. Namely, Claire Plimmer, Stephen Brownlee, Abbie Headon. Extra special thanks to my editor Sophie Martin for your exemplary patience and incisive comments on the structure and focus of the manuscript and to Ray Hamilton for your expert eye for accuracy. To everyone who sponsored us and helped us top £10,000 from the races, quizzes and cake sales, it is helping the MND Association carry on their vital work, thank you. A world free of MND is within reach.

To all the understanding race organisers and charity support – Paul Bond and the Brighton Half Marathon team; Clem Hunnisett and the Martlets Hospice team; Esther Fifield and Sally Light at MND Association; Peter Bryan at Kenilworth Half; Sarah Bland and all at Tempo Events; Andrew Taylor and team at Oxford Half. You removed so many obstacles to make our inclusion possible. You helped us feel like there was no Them and Us.

Thank you to Ruth Osborne for patiently reading the whole manuscript in its early chaotic form and persuading me not to give up. I kept going and look what happened! Also to Sam Staley, Meryl Stanley and Rebecca Pridham for your helpful feedback too.

To those in the public eye who have actively supported us on social media, national radio and with personal messages – especially Jo Pavey, Zoe Ball, Nicky Campbell and Nell McAndrew.

Thanks also to my brother Mark – the finest poet I know – who many years ago helped me believe in the power of my own words. Thank you bro. And to those who spurred me on to write over the years: Steve Lowton (your encouragement was such a turning point), Pete Gilbert (I still have your email from more than a decade ago encouraging me to write a book and get it published), to Jeff Lucas and Rob Parsons, who gave me time and wise advice. And to Tim Robson, who always has a phrase (and a text message) which my head and heart need to hear. Chapeau Tim. You're all heroes in disguise.

Finally to my mum, grandparents and David – you all profoundly shaped my life, including as a runner and as a writer, although you never knew me as one. You're not forgotten.

ABOUT THE AUTHOR

Chris Spriggs is a runner (in denial about getting slower), writer and coach. He is the founder and director of the mentoring charity Lifespace Trust and a coach with NowShowUp.com. He lives near Stratford-upon-Avon with his triathlete wife and three children (all of whom are getting faster). Chris has spoken on local and national radio, and written for a number of national magazine publications, including *Men's Running* and *Youthwork*.

You can follow him on Twitter at @ThinkSmileRun and he keeps a blog at www.thinksmilerun.blogspot.com

Contact details:
Motor Neurone Disease Association
PO Box 246, Northampton, NN1 2PR
Tel: 01604 250505
Email: enquiries@mndassociation.org
Website: www.mndassociation.org
Twitter: @mndassoc

Other resources:
Parkrun: www.parkrun.org.uk
Brighton Marathon: www.brightonmarathon.co.uk
Lifespace Trust: www.lifespace.org.uk

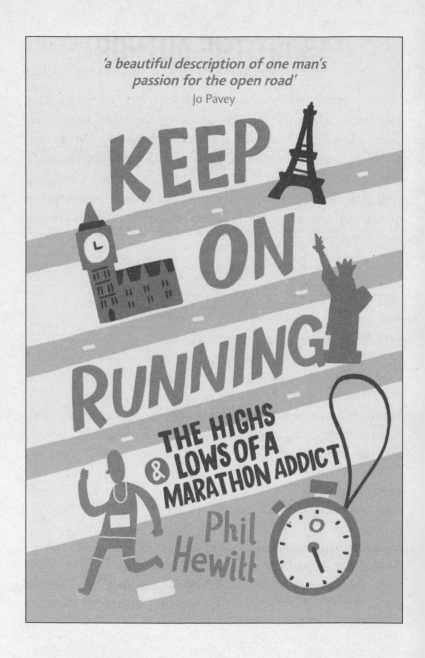

*'a beautiful description of one man's
passion for the open road'*
Jo Pavey

KEEP

ON

RUNNING

THE HIGHS
& LOWS OF A
MARATHON ADDICT

Phil Hewitt

KEEP ON RUNNING
The Highs and Lows of a Marathon Addict

Phil Hewitt

ISBN: 978 1 84953 236 5   Paperback   £8.99

Marathons make you miserable, but they also give you the most unlikely and the most indescribable pleasures. It's a world that I love – a world unlocked when you dress up in lycra, put plasters on your nipples and run 26.2 miles in the company of upwards of 30,000 complete strangers.

Phil Hewitt, who has completed over 25 marathons in conditions ranging from blistering heat to snow and ice, distils his personal experiences into a light-hearted account of his adventures along the way from Berlin to New York, and explores our growing fascination with marathon running. This story of an ordinary guy's addiction to running marathons – an addiction hundreds of thousands share – looks at the highs and lows, the motivation that keeps you going when your body is crying out to stop, and tries to answer the ultimate question, 'Why do you do it?'

'A wonderful and frank view of a first-time-marathoner-turned-running-addict'

Liz Yelling, double Olympian and
Commonwealth bronze medallist

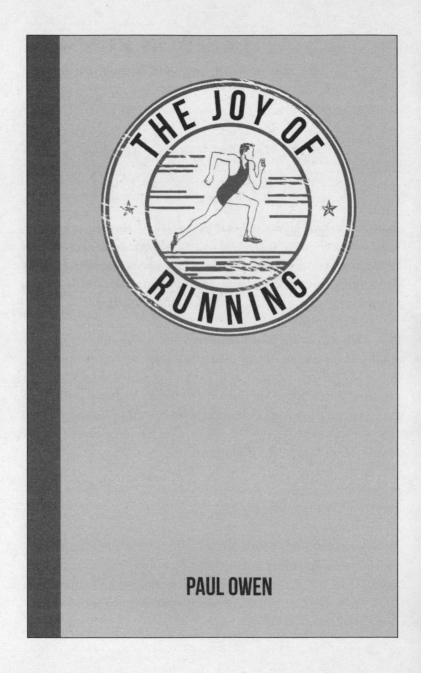

THE JOY OF
RUNNING

PAUL OWEN

THE JOY OF RUNNING
For Those Who Love to Run

Paul Owen

ISBN: 978 1 84953 458 1   Hardback   £9.99

This pocket-sized miscellany, packed with fascinating facts, handy hints and captivating stories and quotes from the world of running, is perfect for anyone who knows the incomparable joy and freedom of lacing up your trainers and hitting the road.

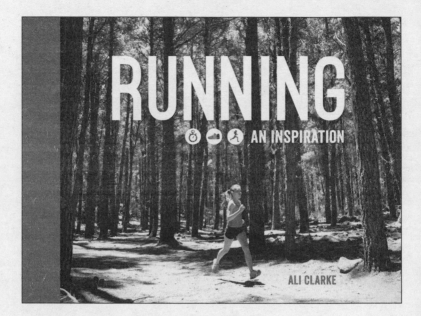

RUNNING

AN INSPIRATION

ALI CLARKE

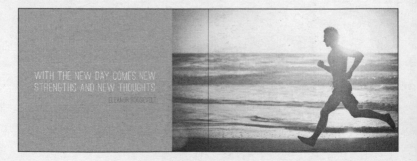

WITH THE NEW DAY COMES NEW
STRENGTHS AND NEW THOUGHTS
ELEANOR ROOSEVELT

RUNNING
An Inspiration

Ali Clarke

ISBN: 978 1 84953 615 8   Hardback   £14.99

Running isn't a hobby, it's a way of life. Capturing the strength, the speed, the stamina and the pure exhilaration of a great run, these stunning photographs and inspiring quotations showcase the beauty of the world's most enduringly popular sport.

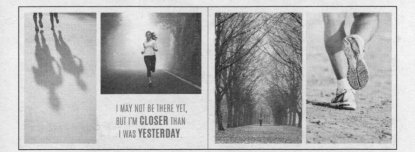

I MAY NOT BE THERE YET, BUT I'M **CLOSER** THAN I WAS **YESTERDAY**.

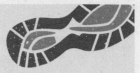

'Practical, encouraging and funny –
the ideal guide for women looking
to get into triathlon'
Kate Carter, *The Guardian*

TRICURIOUS

Surviving the Deep End, Getting into Gear and Racing to Triathlon Success

Laura Fountain
and Katie King

TRICURIOUS
Surviving the Deep End, Getting into Gear and Racing to Triathlon Success

Laura Fountain & Katie King

ISBN: 978 1 84953 714 8   Paperback   £8.99

Laura was a self-certified couch potato who, until a few years ago, could only run for a couple of minutes at a time, and couldn't swim. She has now completed several marathons and is a committed triathlete.

But Laura couldn't have achieved what she has without the advice and support of her friend Katie. A life-long runner, fair-weather cyclist and born-again swimmer, Katie helped Laura through the ups and downs of training for a triathlon. As well as surmounting fears of failure and, more importantly, Laura's fears of drowning in the swim start, their triathlon journey gave them the opportunity to push their limits and have fun along the way.

Tricurious tells Laura's and Katie's story with energy and humour. Filled with anecdotes and advice about the trials and tribulations of preparing for a triathlon, this inspiring book will answer your questions and leave you curious to experience the joy (and pain) of swim, bike, run.

Have you enjoyed this book?
If so, why not write a review on your favourite website?

If you're interested in finding out more about our books,
find us on Facebook at **Summersdale Publishers** and follow
us on Twitter at **@Summersdale**.

Thanks very much for buying this Summersdale book.

www.summersdale.com